Advance praise for JoAnneh Nagler and *Naked Marriage*

"Nagler infuses exquisite sensitivity with courageous honesty in this wise counsel about the most intimate matters confronted in marriage. Rather than a guidebook for *falling* in love, *Naked Marriage* implores the willingness necessary for *staying* in love."

—Rabbi Peter J. Rubinstein, Director of Jewish Community and Bronfman Center for Jewish Life, 92nd Street Y

"Although a plethora of books offer the alluring but ultimately false promise of eternal marital bliss, Nagler actually delivers a sensible, engaging, and remarkably pleasurable blueprint for creating intimacy in our long-term relationships."

—David A. Levy, professor of psychology, Pepperdine University

"Nagler tells us how to stay close and intimate in simple, direct, easy-to-put-into-practice suggestions which really work. I recommend this book to everyone who wants their long-term relationship to remain satisfyingly wonderful. Ms. Nagler will show you that hers has, and yours can, too."

—Isadora Alman, MFT, CST, author of
What People Keep Asking Me About Sex and Relationships

"Having been an attorney for over thirty-five years in the world of family law and the dissolution of marriages, I found Nagler's book to provide pro-active and provocative tools for couples who want to rediscover and sustain a relationship full of devotion, respect, kindness, and life-long love."

—Amy Rodney, family law attorney

"*Naked Marriage* exposes our most intimate vulnerabilities and then leads us to a warm, non-threatening instruction on sensual partnership. We all know the challenges we face in marriage, so I deeply appreciated JoAnneh's step-by-step approach, keeping strategies simple and offering personalized, loving assistance. Though the book focuses on intimacy, many of the practices will work for other life challenges, too, but probably best to wear clothes for those. I loved this book!"

—Samantha Krawitzky, MD

NAKED MARRIAGE

HOW TO HAVE A LIFETIME OF LOVE, SEX, JOY, AND HAPPINESS

JOANNEH NAGLER

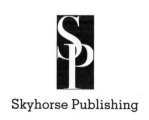

Skyhorse Publishing

Skyhorse Publishing books may be purchased in bulk at special discounts for sales promotion, corporate gifts, fund-raising, or educational purposes. Special editions can also be created to specifications. For details, contact the Special Sales Department, Skyhorse Publishing, 307 West 36th Street, 11th Floor, New York, NY 10018 or info@skyhorsepublishing.com.

Skyhorse® and Skyhorse Publishing® are registered trademarks of Skyhorse Publishing, Inc.®, a Delaware corporation.

Visit our website at www.skyhorsepublishing.com.

10 9 8 7 6 5 4 3 2 1

Library of Congress Cataloging-in-Publication Data

Names: Nagler, JoAnneh, author.
Title: Naked marriage: how to have a lifetime of love, sex, joy, and
    happiness / JoAnneh Nagler.
Description: New York, NY: Skyhorse Publishing, [2018]
Identifiers: LCCN 2017058358 | ISBN 9781510733596 (hardcover: alk. paper)
Subjects: LCSH: Sex in marriage. | Sex. | Intimacy (Psychology) | Married
    people—Sexual behavior. | Married people—Psychology.
Classification: LCC HQ31 .N245 2018 | DDC 306.7--dc23 LC record available
    at https://lccn.loc.gov/2017058358

Cover design by Jane Sheppard
Cover photo credit: iStockphoto

Print ISBN: 978-1-5107-3359-6
Ebook ISBN: 978-1-5107-3360-2

Printed in the United States of America

For Michael: for your devotion, your faith in me,
and your willingness to build our marriage with passion
and adoration as its guiding stars.

CONTENTS

PREFACE

My husband and I have been married twice—to each other. Two weddings, two marriages, and two very different experiences of being in love.

When we married the first time we ran our ship aground on many of the usual things that make a marriage fail: we couldn't communicate our needs in a constructive way; our money and debt issues pressed us into a corner with each other (which made us feel trapped); our sex life deteriorated; and we began to feel boxed in, misunderstood, and hurt.

We thought we were going to be different from all of the other troubled couples in the world. We hated to fight and hated to raise our voices, so we just avoided the hard subjects. Issues with sex, money, affection, time, how we were communicating, and our life choices all got swept under the rug. We knew we loved each other, so why rock the boat?

The times we attempted to talk to each other about what wasn't working disintegrated into stand-offs. I would bring up an issue in the worst way: speaking like a therapist and making pronouncements about what we should do. My husband would shut down and literally not speak to me for days. The message I heard from his silence: *If you want me to love you, don't bring up that subject.* Since avoidance was a dynamic in both of our upbringings, we were perfectly poised for the poison of that stance to ruin us.

We had no capacity to look difficulty in the face, to turn its dimensions over in our hands, to ruminate on it long enough to thoughtfully come up with a productive next step. And when that began to affect our intimacy, we had no strategies to return to each other when our ship started taking water over the side.

Our sex life started to suffer. We couldn't come to each other with respect and ease and freedom, so we were at odds. I would press for more sex, believing that would solve our distances, and my husband would resist me, feeling the weight of my desperation.

After three years of living together and four years of marriage, we were heading into a divorce.

We separated, and I moved four hundred miles away. Over the next several years, we saw each other dozens of times, trying to make our relationship re-cement itself with sexual experiences and long-distance longing, but we were getting no closer to solving what needed to be solved.

We both went out into the world and tried to date, tried to have relationships with other people. But we kept coming back to the love we had for each other, to the inexorable desire to talk to or see each other. It was an excruciating ping-pong ball experience for both of our hearts, and it ended with us vowing never to speak to one another again.

Then something changed. We both became willing. Maybe it was recognizing how truly rare and amazing it is to be completely drawn to another human being; to love and trust another person over time. Maybe it was a bit of wisdom that came with being older. Certainly, there were some practical things. I had to learn to live within my means and still be able to explore my creative life. He had to make peace with the way he chose to live in the world—as a teacher and an activist—and be willing to fund his life with the cash he had, not adding the weighty pressure of borrowing to the mix. And we both had to learn to speak up, even about difficult things.

One day, several years after our divorce, I invited him to lunch. "What the hell," he said, "let's have dinner." We did and had a terrific time. When I got back home he called and said, "We've been here for each other for better or worse—even through a divorce—and I want to try getting back together." I paused, took a big breath, and said, "Okay. Let's go to therapy."

After about twenty minutes the therapist looked at us and said, "I've got couples who are much worse off than you two are and they're making it, so what's the holdout?"

So, we got back together. We made some promises: when there was trouble, we would come towards the relationship, not move away from it—meaning we had to be willing to talk. We would live within our means. We both had to figure out a simple way to manage our lives, our time, our money—together and individually—and we had to do it without micromanaging the other.

Then the real work began. Neither one of us had had a regular sex life for a while and didn't know how to move back into a steady intimacy. We had no idea what our needs were for regular and frequent affection, communication, and expressions of love. Since both of us had things we loved to do in the world beyond our day jobs, we had issues with time.

There were past dating partners who would call looking for a hit of intrigue; friends who were used to us being single and resented our newly imposed relationship focus, and a whole slew of new extended family issues that we had to deal with.

We had to build paths, bridges, and roads, to find our way over or around every one of those obstacles. It wasn't easy. It was a hand-to-hand climb up a rocky, slippery traverse, with no guideposts, no road signs, no storybook bread crumb trail appearing through the wild weeds that kept whacking us in the face.

I remember being in our flat's tiny kitchen in a deep knee bend with my butt up against the refrigerator as I was trying to get to the broiler, and then burning my forearm on the oven. I ran barefoot out of the apartment yelling, "I can't do this!"

My husband chased me down, took me gently by the shoulders, and said, "Come back. Please!" I did. In that small moment we found a little bit of the magic dust that makes a marriage work: *willingness*. We didn't have the answers. We didn't have any ideas for solving some of our problems, but we were *willing*. That changed everything. Over the next few years, we had to overcome the death traps and land mines from our first marriage. We had to figure out who we are now and build something together based on that. We had to listen to what the other was moved by and not moved by.

We had to notice that no matter what the culture is babbling on about regarding relationships, it's ultimately just me and him—two frail-hearted and quirky individuals with needs and desires, gifts and graces—who will either build a road in the middle together or not.

We built that road, he and I. I wrote this book about some of the things we learned in our second-time-around marriage, our love affair that has been reclaimed from the junk heap and now gleams and shines and zips around in the world, full of delight and joy.

Because I had no real help or strategies our first time around—and we had no solid strategies together—I lost many years with the husband I love. Though I am grateful for our happiness now, sometimes I miss those years. I would have liked very much to have had some simple ideas thrown our way, some skills offered, and some learning tools planted in our path that might have helped us find our way *before* we got into terrible trouble.

More than anything else, this book is about the willingness to do something *now*; to not have to go to the brink of divorce before we're willing to learn the skills that will help us be happier and closer. It's about learning how to be a good partner—a giving, sensual, and intimate one—over the course of years. It's a book of easy-to-apply shortcuts that can help each of us experience a full and grateful-for-it-every-hour marriage. It's the guidebook that would have helped keep us from floundering and falling down the first time around.

Though our path was one of dissolution and restoration, this book is not designed to address couples who are in total breakdown. It is not a therapy-based book, and does not seek to cover every aspect of adult marital experience.

Instead, it's a book about intimacy and creating it. It's a guide for couples who know they love each other and want to stay close, but have found it difficult to create the ways, the willingness, or the time for regular closeness.

Intimacy is so much more than just sensual contact. It's also about being able to talk to each other, make decisions together—particularly about money, family, and lifestyle—and share fun and romantic moments. These things support our unobstructed sensual and sexual intimacy, so *Naked Marriage* offers straightforward strategies on how to get to those things as well, with simple shortcuts that we can apply right now, without digging up the past.

The ideas on these pages provide a kick-start, a box full of things to try in your life and marriage to see if they make your heart rumble and your body tingle, and then make you willing. It's a book of loving suggestions and ideas—a start-from-today, take-what-you-like-and-leave-the-rest approach—that can help you deepen your delight with your partner, or come back to your partner if you've been distant.

It's about learning some easy skills that will help us all *love well over time*, offering the tactile, sensuous experience of a "forever love," in the best sense of the phrase.

The suggestions I share in this book have made my marriage work, making it a happy place to dwell. I hope you will find within these pages the reclamation of joy and desire that my husband and I have found; the blessing of a true, lasting, and passionate love affair.

May marital love and devotion grace your doorstep, and find a sensual home in your heart, your body, your bed, and your spirit.

—JoAnneh Nagler

INTRODUCTION

One day I woke up and realized that life is never going to get calm and quiet enough for us married people to have a free and easy intimate life. While we're dating we rush toward our partner with open hearts and bodies, freely throwing aside anything we can run away from to get back into our lover's arms. We're breathless with adoration and heat for our partner, and we can't wait to dive back in to the sweet and sweaty intimacies of being with each other.

Then we get married. We put our lot in with the person we most respect, most long for, and most hold dear and begin to build a life.

Slowly, over the course of that building, we're pulled and shoved by the pressures of all kinds of outside stuff. Responsibilities. Duties. Unexpected calls upon our time. Disasters and emergencies both inside and outside our family unit that steal away our intimate moments. The passion that had us drop everything to be in the arms of our lover is smothered.

Beyond duties and outside angst, we also have the pressures from all the stuff that comes up *between* us. How to live our lives. What lifestyle choices to make. Where we should live. How to handle our money. Kids. How to field involvement from each other's parents and natal family.

And there's always a wrench being thrown into the works. We may not have been raised with healthy communication skills, so we can't now—in our marriage—negotiate the land of expressing our needs

and thoughts at all, or without agitation. We may not know how to
bring up a difficult subject if we know we'll disagree with our partner.
We may not have any language at all for talking about sex and affection, or know how to ask for what we want in that area.

Many of us find that sex and sensuality, after all of the other calls
upon our time in a given week, end up taking a back seat. They sit on
the shelf, sidelined day after day behind all of the other "important"
things that demand our attention. They drift. And so we drift away
from each other. We become roommates instead of lovers.

Many of us don't have the skills necessary for being intimate *over
time*. Meaning, we don't know how to access our desire, or spark it.
We know, though, by looking around at the people who've done it
well—who are now well into their marital years and who still adore
each other—that there's nothing sweeter on this earth. *Nothing*.

We know that having a beautiful marriage is a sky's-the-limit, heart-
deepening, thrilling, and worthy cause, worth every bit of effort. Yet,
because we are unschooled in loving over the course of years, we often
flounder. Even with our best intentions face-front in our heart, we
screw up. And we don't screw up because we're just insensitive jerks
who can't get past our own selfishness. (At least that's true for most of
us.) We drive what was once a shiny new car into the junk heap for
one simple reason: *we don't know how to love well over time*.

Marriage is about the long-term. It's about loving over days and
months and years. If we are unschooled in the practice of passion and
closeness over the course of years, we are going to drift apart. We are
going to lose the bright spark of love that drew us together in the first
place, and we will unintentionally take stances of duty, obligation, and
distance with each other.

But here's the good news: we can learn how to have a *practice* of
love, a regular expression of it. In intimacy, in affection, in sex, in
communication, in lifestyle and family choices—in *all* of it. As adults,
even entrenched in old marital habits, we can learn this. And here's the
best part: learning this does not have to be difficult.

Most of us, if we're honest about it, want to be adored and held dear in our love life. We want to reach that twentieth, or thirty-second, or forty-fifth wedding anniversary and be able to say, "She's the love of my life, and I can't possibly imagine a day without her," or "He's the very best person I know, and I am so lucky to be in love with him." We want intimacy, we want sweetness and joy, and we want a grace-filled experience of love.

But look around. Who has taught us to love well? Who has given us the skills we need to help make our genuine commitment translate itself into a daily loving practice? For many of us, the answer is: *no one.* No one has taught us how to do this, so we must teach ourselves.

I decided to write about marriage versus dating and "being in relationships" because marriage is, I believe, where a particular kind of intimacy happens. It's the place where a long-term commitment has been forged and, therefore, can be worked with. In other words, our commitment is a big rock that we can stand upon to deepen our experience with another human being in love.

When I began writing this book, I asked my husband, "How do I share what I want to share without sounding too directive? I don't want the suggestions I'm writing down to sound like a list of therapist's directions to dutifully check off. I want people to be able to use this book to *discover* things—love, regular sensuality, and communication, and the payoff of that, intimately, as a couple."

Then he reminded me of a moment early on in our first marriage, when we were first making a life together. We walked to our local 7–11 to get some juice, and when we were on our way out of the store, a guy we passed said something that just cracked us up. We sat down on a tire stop in the parking lot—tears running down our faces from the hilariousness of it—and could not, for the life of us, stop laughing. Neither of us can remotely remember what was so funny, but we remember that moment as the shift in our loving, when we first honestly relaxed with each other and began to trust. Right then we started to get loose with each other.

Later, when things went awry, we lost that ability. Instead, we were tense and testing, watchful and dissatisfied, waiting for the next shoe to drop between us. That killed our ease with each other, as well as our sex life.

Now, in our second marriage, after using so many of the suggestions we'll be talking about in this book, we have found that lightness again, and it has lasted. That speaks to my original question to my husband about this book's tone. I'm not offering the suggestions in this book to help us be good little marital citizens. I'm not offering them as a to-do list, to be checked off so that we "get it right." I'm sharing these things because in my own marriage I found that when we returned to intimacy we were able to relax with each other once more. Our good humor returned, and we started feeling free with each other again—just like that night on the tire stop outside the convenience store.

The best thing we can bring to our marriage is *willingness*. We have to love our partner enough to be willing to try to make our experience together more peaceful, more honest, more courageous, more open-hearted, and more sensual. To bring our A game to the table and start taking steps to play it out. I truly believe that the skills of loving well can be learned, simply and easily—and that, in fact, they *need* to be learned. That's why I've crafted this book.

We once loved our partner more than life itself and could hardly hold our breath in our chest for wanting more passionate moments with our lover. That exhilarating openness, more mature now and grounded upon a foundation of years of life experience together, is what we're after.

There is nothing in all of my wild and vast living experience like the grace of being in love. To be in love over time, over days and years, is like slipping into a sensual looking glass of life's sweetest gift. I hope this book helps you find that looking glass—a vision of what enduring passion looks like. May it help you build a home there, grounded in closeness and devotion, filled with the thrill of adoring each other always.

CHAPTER ONE
NAKED DATE

It's hard to have a regular intimate life. We're busy. We've got jobs, families, obligations, community commitments, and bodies that need exercise and rest. We've got homes to attend to. Money issues to field. We've got stuff to maintain and duties to perform: meals to cook, house and yard work, kids' sports practices and school stuff.

Then we've got the things that life throws at us: a parent who is ill, a child with learning disorders, a testy boss, a job loss. We've got deadlines and pressures and problems, along with the need for some kind of creative exploration. On top of all of that, we're probably feeling that we're not earning enough, that somehow we're supposed to be working harder or more.

Then there's the stupid stuff that happens: the car breaks down in the middle of nowhere and it's a five-day wait for the part to arrive to fix the damn thing; the electrical wiring in the house has fried to a crisp so the walls are torn up and the house is a construction zone; a case of bronchial pneumonia makes it impossible to get out of bed for a week.

How on God's green earth are we supposed to maintain an amorous life with our partners through all of that? How can we make time for each other on a regular basis that consists of more than just falling into a heap of exhaustion in front of the flat-screen?

Everyone who has ever been married knows the pull of all this stuff and the effect it has on our love lives. Busyness, stress, and worry, distraction, exertion, and exhaustion drain the passion out of us. They can leave us flat and disinterested in each other, resistant, and too tired for anything remotely sensual.

But there's a way to hold on to our joy. We can learn to *claim* our closeness with our partners—to push back against the world's duties and pressures and insist upon our time together.

A little bit of time each and every week is all we're after. Enough to reconnect, to keep our desire alive and well, and to escape from life's stresses and obligations long enough to *let go into each other.*

That doesn't sound like too much to ask for from a marriage, does it? It's *not.* But how do we manage that? *We get ourselves a Naked Date.*

What's a Naked Date?

The Naked Date is an hour or two we set aside each week to get naked with each other. It's a set time that allows us to take off our clothes, get in bed, and get close to each other. It might be sexual; it might not be. It is *scheduled sensual time* during which we set aside the pressures of daily life and get next to each other, skin to skin.

It's ease and grace time, close time, amorous time that lets us find each other again—a practice we engage in, slowly and deliberately, to keep our connection strong and alive.

It can be any time we choose, and the only rule is this: it needs to be a time we can honor each and every week. It could be Tuesday evenings at seven, when the kids are at basketball practice. It could be Sunday night at six, when we have no other obligations. It could be Saturday morning at eight, when the rest of the family is still asleep.

The only guiding principle of using the Naked Date is this: *you must choose a time you can honor each and every week.*

In my marriage, we chose Friday nights at six. That means we don't make plans. It means our extended family knows we don't get together on Friday nights. It means we stop what we're doing at five or five thirty and get ready to be together.

The Naked Date is not a time to vent about your controlling boss or discuss your child's learning disability; it's not the time to banter about the repairs going on in the kitchen or whether you should put your house on the market. In fact, it's not a talking event at all. In its purest form, the Naked Date is a time to get sensual, get skin-to-skin, and be close—a time set aside for love, sex, and intimate sensuality.

Does it have to be sexual every time? No. But it does need to be *close*. Many couples find that quiet, intimate, naked time together will lead to some kind of sexual closeness. But the object, every time, is to get close for an uninterrupted hour or two to reconnect.

What we need is a little bit of time, each and every week—enough time to keep our adult passion alive and well and to escape from the stresses and obligations long enough to *let go and find some delight together.*

How it works

You'll set a time—say, Sunday night at seven—when each of you must be in bed, naked. Again, the time doesn't matter; what does matter is that you choose a regular time—an hour in which you won't be interrupted; a set time you can come back to each and every week.

Ten minutes before your time, you'll want to turn your attention away from phones, devices, errands, and duties. Don't start doing "this one little thing." Don't start dinner or rake the yard or take a bath. You want to be ready for your partner at the time you specified. When you do this week after week, your partner will begin to feel the respect you offer him or her by your willingness to show up. He or she will know that you value your intimate time together, and that you're willing to set aside your worries and cares and then *connect*. That's a huge thing all by itself.

The Naked Date is about sensing—it's not about imposing anything on one another. It's about feeling into each other's skin and breath and heart. It's about finding a sensual expression of your love. *Be naked and be close.* That's the idea. Listen for your partner's body signals. Listen for his or her breath, for what makes your partner truly fall into your arms.

There's vulnerability and an openness that occurs when we lie together without clothes on—it's as if that very act helps us throw off the world's responsibilities for an hour or so, and that's usually all we need to sense and feel the ease that comes from being close to our partners. Whether we're sexual or not, we want to hold each other and be close for at least an hour.

The Naked Date is a shortcut to intimacy—we're using a set time to make sure that no matter what else happens during the week, we will get the regular experience of being close. Its regularity is its gift. We don't have to think about whether our partner wants us enough or whether or not we have the courage to approach them. We don't have to worry about whether or not we will connect or get sensual and be close. It's already set up, and all we have to do to get there is show up. That's the magic of the Naked Date. All it takes to own and experience our intimacy every week is a little reframing of our thought processes and a willingness to try something new.

That's the idea.

Marriage is a different animal than dating

Why do we need a Naked Date? Can't we just get naked spontaneously when the mood strikes us both? No. And here's why.

Marriage is not a spontaneous animal. Marital life does not lend itself to the kind of random sexuality and closeness that populated our dating lives. More often than not, we drift in marriage from week to week with no sensual contact whatsoever—not out of a lack of love, but from being beaten down by life's responsibilities and time pressures.

I interviewed many couples when writing this book, and no matter how close to their spouse they reported feeling, *each and every partner* said that it is "difficult," "challenging," "tough," and sometimes, "like climbing a mountain" to just carve out a little time for closeness and sensual contact.

We drift. We don't mean to, but we do. We know we love each other, but somehow we don't find the time to be intimate, and we make excuses: the mood isn't right, one of us is too tired, one of us has had a terrible week. So desire drifts as well, and we begin to lose the need to find each other amorously and erotically that we once had.

Our cultural mores sometimes get in the way, too. Many images of marriage in popular culture show it as something that loses desire over time. We've been told again and again—through movies, books, TV, as well as our "conventional wisdom"—that marital desire loses its luster. So many of us have grown up accepting the idea of dwindling desire in marriage without thinking twice about it. We don't have an adult model for healthy intimacy, and we don't think of long-term loving as a deepening of desire.

We begin to slip away from each other, and it hurts.

What we want more than anything in marriage is to experience the love we have—to revel in it, to claim it over years. We want to do more than know that we love our partner; we want to *feel* it.

So we need an hour or two each week to throw off the world's duties and disappear into the release and ease that brought us together in the first place.

The Naked Date is how we get there.

Anneke and Jonathan

Anneke and Jonathan were new parents with an eight-month-old son when we first spoke. Contrary to the experience of some new moms who lose interest in sex for a while, Anneke's experience had heightened her sexual desire.

"I feel like I'm so completely in love with my son that I could just explode with it," she said. "I don't know why, but the whole thing has made me feel completely sexually electrified. But it seems like I always want it in the daytime, and Jonathan wants it late at night—if he wants it at all—so we end up never doing it."

Being a new parent was pulling Jonathan in a different direction. "Family is where my focus is," he explained. "And since Anneke's and my body cycles seem to be literally night and day, it seems like too much work to pursue it that hard."

When we talked about trying a Naked Date to help curb disappointed expectations and the pressure to have sex, both partners balked.

"I don't want to be forced to have sex with my wife because I'm supposed to," Jonathan said. Anneke winced. "Wow. That makes me feel like crap, Jon. You really don't want to make an effort to be with me at all do you?"

Rather than go down that rocky road of airing what each was feeling, I suggested they try a strategy to help shift their *behavior* for the good of their marriage. I call it "The Science Experiment" approach.

I explained how the Naked Date works to create a habit in our minds and bodies that allows us to prepare for intimacy, providing a bit of ramp up to get ready to let our guard down. It also helps tremendously with frequency expectations.

Anneke said, "I seriously could have sex every day right now. I know this won't last, but that's how I feel."

In response, Jonathan said, "I just can't live up to that kind of pressure."

They needed a strategy to meet in the middle and also had to address the issue of *when* to be intimate. Anneke is dead tired late at night after working and taking care of their son and tries to go to bed early. Jonathan gets a second wind after nine o'clock, and that's when he gets relaxed enough to think about sex.

Based on these challenges, I invited them to try meeting up intimately on Sundays at four p.m. and dedicate an hour to getting naked. Sunday was family dinner night at Anneke's aunt's house (a ten-minute drive away), so their strategy was to drop off their son early at her aunt's, then return home for some naked time, then head back for dinner at six thirty.

However, they quickly figured out that when they both dropped off the baby they became engaged in the family conversation, little to-do's, and efforts to help. Then Jonathan would say, "We're already here, so we might as well just stay." As a result, Anneke would be hurt and angry.

The solution: Anneke dropped off the baby by herself and had her aunt come out to the car to take him, then she zipped right back home. Jonathan agreed to try to settle himself during that time—not making phone calls or answering emails or texts, but just getting still and thinking about something sensual so he'd genuinely prepare.

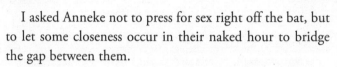

I asked Anneke not to press for sex right off the bat, but to let some closeness occur in their naked hour to bridge the gap between them.

It worked. After a few weeks, they got their sexual groove back. They agreed that if Anneke needed more sexual satisfaction than their weekly Naked Date, she would take care of herself in some solo pleasure, taking the pressure off Jonathan.

They also agreed that if they missed their Naked Date for any reason, they would make it up by setting another time within forty-eight hours. That way Anneke could relax and know that she'd still get to have some sex and intimacy with her husband, and Jonathan would know when so he could prepare.

After two months, Jonathan said, "We're keeping the four o'clock Sundays. But what's better is that if for some reason the whole thing falls apart, like one week we had to take our son to the urgent care, I find myself looking for another time to make love with her right away, and then I really look forward to it."

Anneke was visibly and emotionally relieved. "I think doing it every week on our Naked Dates, and then having some space in between, has made me pay attention to how much I love and look forward to having sex with Jon. Now I want the anticipation, too, almost as much as the act!"

Intimacy requires slow, steady quiet time

When we fall in love it's as if we're on an island—just the two of us—and the whole world has faded into the backdrop—a pale and fading faux scenery that has no claim on our time or our interest. We are quite literally *in love*. We are in the swoon of it, carried on the wings of it, in the altered state of it, and the land of the pedantic, duty-bound world is so distant from our high-in-the-sky view that we can barely make out where we used to stand upon its surface.

But marriage changes that. We become something more than lovers. We fulfill bigger roles: parenting, earning, building a place in our communities. In other words, we contribute to things larger than our own one-on-one partnership.

So it's easy to begin to primarily identify as a couple with the external things we do, with the contributions we make that are sanitized, if you will, for public viewing. And when we do that we can lose track of our private selves, and then begin to lose the sexual intimacies that bring us closer to each other and solidify our bond.

Intimacy in marriage requires slow, steady, quiet time that allows us to focus our desire on our partner. The Naked Date offers us time to be still long enough to hear the pangs of desire inside ourselves and inside our lover. It allows us time to remember that we *are* lovers first and foremost, and then it gives us room to give up our daytime selves so we can slip back into our intimate natures.

We know that we feel better when we connect intimately with each other. We know that being close, touching, making love, having a good romp—and doing it regularly—is good for our marriage.

We also know that our jam-packed lives are never going to slow down long enough to offer open-ended hours to get that time. If we want amorousness, and passion, and closeness in any form, we have to claim it. We have to plan for it, set it up, show up, and take it.

That's why we need a Naked Date.

Give up the myth of spontaneity

The first thing that marriage partners always say to me when I talk about using the Naked Date is this: "Well, that's just not spontaneous enough for me. I can't just turn a switch at an allotted hour and get in the mood."

But the truth is we actually can. We can train ourselves—on Fridays at six, Thursdays at ten, or Sunday mornings at eight—to be available sensually to ourself and our partner. In fact, we *want* to train our bodies and minds to wake up sexually and sensually at a particular time.

Why? Because when we develop that sense of a specific time cue, it's like a clock that ticks us into awareness each week and lets us know that it's time to set aside the world's worries and entanglements and engage in some fulfilling intimacy with the person we love best. The set time—the Naked Date—becomes our cue for loving.

Researchers Benjamin Saunders and Terry Robinson at the University of Michigan (http://ow.ly/y1j33049eVp) studied motivational cues and reported: "We are just beginning to understand the factors . . . in which reward cues acquire powerful motivational properties, and therefore, the ability to act as incentive stimuli." In other words, when we develop a cue, or what psychologists call a "conditioned stimulus," that cue has the power to activate complex emotional and motivational states. In plain English, that means we can thoughtfully create a strong cue for a particular positive purpose, which in this case is *to get close to our partner on a regular basis.*

The key word in that last sentence is *regular.* Sure, spontaneity kicks in once in a while in marriage. But if we are waiting for random acts of intimacy to occur in perfectly aligned mutual desire, we are going to be waiting a long time. If we're holding on to the myth of falling into bed together when the stars are perfectly aligned, we'll end up stealing intimate time from our partnership.

Sadly, that's what many of us have been doing—robbing ourselves of the joy we deserve by insisting that it occur as a spontaneous act.

What if we gave up insisting that our sensuality be spontaneous and showed up for what we say is important to us? What if we stopped thinking that sex in marriage should look the way it did when we were dating? What if we had a strategy, a simple shortcut to help us get next to each other each week, which provides the sensual space to relax and explore each other?

That doesn't sound like too much to ask for the good of our marriage, does it?

It *isn't*. And that's what the Naked Date gives us, each and every week.

Be willing to shift your perspective

In order to make this thing work, we have to be willing to shift our perspective. We have to give up the myth that spontaneity is the only real way to find fulfillment together; that falling into bed suddenly and impulsively is the only genuine way to get to the good stuff.

Most of us have been brought up with next to no training on how to be a good lover, so we have nothing much to go on when we're trying to forge a passionate bond with our partner. But the one thing that many of us got out of our early sexual experiences was this: we believe that intimacy needs to rise up from inside us and take us over so intensely that we run through the wheat fields toward each other, tearing our clothes off and landing in a heap, limbs akimbo.

And that's amazing when it happens. But a long-term marriage asks much more of us than those rare moments of sexual hunger. Marriage is about *loving over time.* It's about digging in to a life together, and for most of us that means there's less time for randomness to take us over, and more things that conspire against it.

So we have to fight back against the things that take away our passion. We have to create time for it and *take it,* so we get to have our amorousness each and every week, no matter what else is going on.

When I first proposed the Naked Date to my husband, he said, "I couldn't do that! It's too structured, and it's way too much pressure." And I get that. But I realized spontaneity was not getting us to be sensual with each other regularly. Without a set time to be together, we were drifting. If there was a stressor during the week for either one of us, we passed on making love. Our schedules are crazy during the week, so, for the most part, weekdays were out; our obligations are heavy, so our conversations tended to focus on them; and our sweet talk deteriorated to a ships-passing-in-the-night information-giving brusqueness.

The Naked Date evolved for us because I could see that we needed some regular time to be together so that if everything went to hell in a handbasket, we could still connect. If we did have some spontaneous sex, well, bravo! But more often than not in our marriage, life was going to interrupt us—it would block our desire, our energy, our willingness, or our time. So we needed to do something about that.

With a bit of willingness, a few simple strategies, and some practice, we were off to the races. Just trying it—taking a stab at having a regular time for intimacy—changed absolutely everything. It opened up a window for having sex and sensuality that made us each relax about *when,* and gave us a little ramp-up time to get ready for the other person's attention. And that relaxed us not only in our sex life, but in every aspect of our marriage.

As I've shared the idea of the Naked Date with other couples (particularly the dozens and dozens of couples I interviewed for this book), those who have tried it have reported the same thing: when they get to their weekly intimacy date, they build the kind of closeness that's joyful and brings ease to their marriage. That's what we want.

A naked love potion

If we've been drifting in distance in our marriages, waiting for random acts of sensuality to connect us, we've probably been experiencing big gaps in the timeline of when we get close and sexual. (This was true for most of the long-time married couples I interviewed.) Trust me when I say that almost none of us know how to connect intimately with our partner regularly over years and years, through slammed schedules, obligations, disappointments, and pressures—and particularly through times when the proverbial roof is caving in and the floodgates have broken open.

We need some straightforward structures to help us. We need a simple, yet flexible, way to find each other intimately on a regular basis, no matter what else is happening. We need a *cue* to help us key in to the fact that it's time to connect, time to be close.

The Naked Date is that cue—a time-specific love potion that trains us to turn our attention to intimacy when everything else would conspire to distract us, like a light switch we can turn to "on" when it's time to get close. I know what you're thinking. You're thinking "Hey! My desire doesn't just switch to 'on' at a set time! I can't get in the mood *on cue.*"

Once again, *yes, you can.* You can train yourself—for the good of your marriage and your own pleasure—to be ready for love at a specific time. Even if you think you can't, you really can. All it takes is a tiny bit of practice, and suddenly your head kicks in and wakes up your body at the appointed hour.

When my husband and I first put the Naked Date into practice he balked at every turn. *Didn't I want to have dinner first? Didn't I feel tired after a long week? Didn't I want to go out to a movie first? Didn't I think this whole thing was way too structured and just too much?* But I held to my request. I wanted to try it and see if it would help us get used to connecting. I wanted to have regular sex with the person I adore. I didn't want our evenings to slide into ten or eleven o'clock at night, when we were beat and exhausted and would postpone our intimacy another week—or two or three. Of all the things I do in a week that I have to "get up" for, this was the thing I most wanted to walk away from my week with: closeness, and love, along with the ease and communion that sensuality with each other brings.

After about two months of trying the Naked Date, we got the hang of it. We had to attempt it, and bottom out, then land at the pizza joint instead, or end up falling asleep at 7:30 after a fifty-hour work week. We had to try it again, and then fail at it again, then try some more until we got it. Now that it's wired into us, we both have an internal clock that starts ticking somewhere around six. If I'm swirling with some work near our appointed time, my husband will say, "Babe. Put that down. It's almost six." And I do. If he's hustling around trying to field emails or emptying the grocery bags, I'll say, "Honey. Leave them. It's six." And then we head off for our naked time.

That's the object: regular, cued, practiced time set aside for each other, *with* each other, each and every week, no matter what.

No matter what

Note that when I say "no matter what," I'm not talking about being unreasonable about sticking to your Naked Date; for instance, if someone in your family has died; if one partner is sick; or if your child has been taken by ambulance to the hospital with a severely broken leg.

When I say *each week, no matter what*, what I mean is that we're not going to beg off from our partner because we're tired or stressed or have had a disappointment. If we use those excuses, we'd never have an intimate life, ever. We're *all* stressed. We're *all* overtired. That's modern life.

That's the reason why we need to test out the time slot for our Naked Date and see if it will work. We need to find the time when we're most willing and likely to show up for the good of our marriage, and then *train* ourselves to do just that.

It's not going to feel easy every time, and it's going to take some effort at the beginning. That's the nature of creating a new habit. But the commitment to show up is what we want to build upon. On the Naked Dates during which we're not at our best, we must *allow and permit* ourselves to be led into love.

That's the gift of having a partner: sometimes they will lead us into love, and sometimes we will lead them. That's how to stay close and loving, near to each other's hearts, alive in our love for each other.

Know that we want to be reasonable and adjustable in emergencies, but we don't want to use the excuse of having a busy life to not try. Remember, it is willingness that builds trust in marriage; it is willingness that has the capacity to build intimacy.

Set a date

When we hold on to the idea that spontaneity is a prerequisite for intimacy, we often go back in our minds to when we were young, to when we were searching and exploring in our dating and sexual lives. And that's fair enough. We remember that it felt thrilling to discover something new—a person we were intrigued with, hot for, or maybe someone we already loved, and then found the thrill of sex with them for the first time. But when we hold our marital sex to that early spontaneity bar, we're really not being honest about how our lives were structured then.

Intimacy in the early days of loving is not really impulsive and unplanned at all. When we were dating, or even "hooking up," we knew when we were going out. We knew we were meeting our date on a Thursday or a Saturday night, or a Friday afternoon. We thought about it during the week, we planned what we were going to wear, we took time getting ready and dressed, and we got our mind around being with the other person. We had a set time, and we had a ramp-up. Occasionally some sexual experience fell out of the sky and landed in our lap, but most of the time part of the thrill of seeing the other person was our passionate anticipation of the event.

That's the kind of ramp-up we're seeking by using the Naked Date. We want a space in our lives that's carved out for love and sensuousness. We want the ability to think about our partner when we're away from him or her, to dream a little about what we might want to do and feel, to anticipate and dwell in the event in our mind and body. To *long* for our partner a bit. To prepare.

In the weeks when our lives take us over and we haven't had a sexual thought for days, and there's been no real anticipation at all, the Naked Date serves us in another way: it wakes us up, and invites us to show up for sensuality even though we haven't been thinking about it—like a surprise sexual experience we didn't expect. The set time reminds us to put our brain on the shelf, and to allow for our body and heart to lead us to pleasure.

I'm inviting you to think of the Naked Date like a real *date,* a time you've set aside to drop out of the world and get a little free, a little wild, and a little open-bodied—just the way you used to, with the added grace of mature intimacy and commitment.

The only way that's going to happen regularly is if you *set a date.* That's the principle we're working with here.

The body knows things

Our resistance will usually pipe up right about now and say, "Wait a minute. Setting a Naked Date with my partner is not going to be like my early dating life. We've known each other too long for that!"

But funnily enough, the body knows things. The body knows when it trusts a partner, and it tends to get itself ready when intimacy with that partner is imminent. Our bodies can lead us to each other. All we have to do is set the time and *be there.*

Just like learning to go to the gym, we can learn to show up for ourself and our partner in love. When we're first learning to work out, the key is to show up at the gym no matter how distracted or resistant we feel. Our only job, really, is to get ourself there—to transport our body to the gym door. And as long as we have a simple set of exercises that we know how to do, once we get there, it's easy to get into it. It sort of takes care of itself once we're inside the building. That's the principle of the Naked Date. Once we set aside time, get naked, and get in bed together, the hard part is over. We've pushed past the resistance that might keep us from being available to love, and we're right there, accessible to it.

The Naked Date helps us get past all of the road barriers we put up, the smoke screens we hide behind, and the ice-caves we surround ourselves with—the stuff that hides our fear that we won't have sex, or the fear that we will, and we'll have to be vulnerable. It's a truism of married life that it's hard sometimes to break through the public roles of our wife and husband duties and obligations, and push past them to our original lover connection. Meaning that intimacy, left to life's own devices, can get bowled over by duty. And duty can close us off to our sensitivity, our wants, and our desires. It can shut off the heart's connection to the senses and gets us all jonesed up on the adrenaline of what has to get done next on the to-do checklist.

But when we show up for our Naked Date, we give our bodies a chance to find sensuality—anticipation, getting ready, feeling some longing, and then the pleasure of the actual acts: the sensitivity of being naked against our lover's skin, the soul-ease of being connected, the hot sweetness of being held and touched, the ramp-up of desire, the electricity of some genuine excitement, and the terrific letting go into the rhythm of sexual pleasure itself.

Sensuality as a couple is good; good for our marriage, good for our spirits, and even good for solidifying our family unit. And the Naked Date is here to help us get to that goodness week in and week out.

The Slow Ramp-up

The thought that we can reclaim or reignite the initial passion we had for each other when we were first dating has been talked about and written about by therapists and authors for a long time. But what I'm up to here is something different.

I believe that "time-in" in our marriage brings familiarity, and though we can strive to bring some mystery into our loving, we are now, after years of it, dealing with a different kind of animal than when we were dating. It's more mature, it's built on life experience as well as sexual experience, and it's broader than just passion.

Not only do we know each other well now, we also know each other's sensual needs and quirks, likes and pleasures—in other words, we believe we know what works and what doesn't. As a couple, we have intimate habits as well as daily life habits.

But just because that dating passion isn't present the same way it once was doesn't mean we're lacking in passion. We have a well of it available to us: it just doesn't look, feel, or taste like it once did, and we don't want it to. It's often a slower ramp-up now, but a more familiar opening. And we can build on that opening sensually. Our knowledge of each other can be the bedrock upon which we build new gifts of *prowess* in our sex life. (We'll talk about prowess in detail later.)

Sometimes we spend way too much time regretting the fact that our passion is not the same as when we first met. When we do that we miss the opportunities present in the ability of knowing our partner *now*, and our opportunity as a couple to build on that.

Having "time-in" with each other is truly what allows the Naked Date to work well. We already know each other, and we already have experience with each other's bodies. We can use the shortcut of the time slot and our naked bodies lying next to each other to jump-start our familiar patterns of being sexual and sensual. And that helps us be intimate regularly.

But just because we know some things about our partner doesn't mean we know everything. Sure, our familiarity is the gift that can get us into our Naked Date without a lot of muss and fuss. And that history is like a rock-solid foundation from which we can build a new exploration.

But there's something else. When we commit to finding ways to deepen our intimacy—like keeping a Naked Date—we get to banish all of the nonsense that says the *hot* part of our relationship was at the beginning.

Who says? What if there's a discovery yet to be had?

If we want long-term closeness with our spouse, we have to ask ourself, *what are the gifts of being deeply inside our sensual intimacy for years?*

We want a road that leads us back to intimacy, time and time again, so that we actually get to experience the loving we say we want.

And what does a regular exploration require? What does prowess require? It requires uninterrupted time, willingness, and regularity. And that's exactly what we're giving ourselves with the Naked Date.

A quick disclaimer

The Naked Date is not designed as a panacea for couples who are having terrible, on-the-brink-of-divorce trouble. Lying in bed together naked or having a weekly sex date is not going to do the trick if the two of you have not spoken honestly for years and years. It's also not going to work if one partner is cheating on the other, or if heavy money pressures, debilitating anger, or entrenched resentments have distanced you so severely that you no longer speak or attempt intimate communication at all. This book is not designed to address that kind of trouble.

Though many of the communication, time, money, and affection tips in this book may be useful if both partners are willing to try them, I do not recommend pressing for a Naked Date if everything in your marriage is dissolving. Pressing for sex as a way to glue yourselves back together when you're faltering never works; it just presses the issues farther into the black hole of denial and makes the hurt worse. Oftentimes, in the moment or later on, it can feel violating to one or both partners.

In other words, it's almost impossible to have honest, trust-building, physical and sexual intimacy when there's an intense breakdown and awfulness is happening. You can't just jump into having a Naked Date or attempt to press the idea on your partner if you're entrenched in terrible trouble.

You have to start, instead, with communication, with creating some shared values, with dealing with the elephants in the room. If you're in terrible marital distress, this book really needs to be read backwards, focusing on the building of shared values and using communication tools rather than the physical and sensual intimacy.

This book is for couples who love each other and know they want to be together, but who need tips and suggestions that will help them deepen their intimacy and closeness across a number of marital challenges and over the course of years.

For example, when my husband and I were married the first time and were avoiding all of the troubling things we needed to talk about—the things that were driving us apart—I thought we could weather our unaddressed issues by gluing ourselves together with more sex. That was backwards thinking. Intimacy is a reflection of our commitment and our love, our delight in the other person, and our clear communication and agreement that we want to be together. Intimacy and good sex grow out of our willingness, not the other way around. Meaning we can't make an unwilling partnership become a healthy one by having more sex. It just won't work.

So please, if you're having on-the-brink trouble or you're in total shutdown, get some outside help, and don't expect the Naked Date to fix those issues. The Naked Date is designed for couples who largely get along and know they want to be married to each other, but who need a little help finding some simple ways to support a regular and deepening intimacy.

Two months to create a habit

Dr. Maxwell Maltz, in a classic observation of his patients (see his book *Psycho-Cybernetics, A New Way to Get More Living Out of Life*, 1989) claimed that it "takes 21 days to form a new habit." And though his thought process has been ingrained in our popular culture by authors and motivational seminar leaders like Tony Robbins and others, the actual science behind behavior change is a bit more in-depth.

Later research by Phillippa Lally, a health psychology researcher at the UK Behavioral Research Center, University College London (*European Journal of Social Psychology*, https://www.ucl.ac.uk/news/

news-articles/0908/09080401) suggests that for a habit to become fully ingrained in us, it actually takes about two months.

And that's good news for us married people. Going back to our research on developing cues, we want a relatively short arc for learning how to be intimate regularly. Yes, the Naked Date is going to take some weeks for both our body and mind to learn it; it's going to take a little time for the habit to become fully ingrained.

During the two months or so it'll take to get used to having a Naked Date, we're going to encounter every form of resistance we've ever had to the idea of keeping a regular time for intimacy.

It means he's going to pipe up at 5:59 and say, "Aren't you hungry? Wouldn't you rather eat first?" and drag her out to the burger joint, then claim he's "too full and too tired" by the time they get back home. It means on Saturday morning at 9:58 she'll say, "I have to make this one phone call first—it'll only take two minutes," and then an hour and a half will go by and the kids will be home from soccer practice. It means that one or both of you is going to be tired or distracted or saddened by some event during the week and will want to beg off. That's the nature of learning how to use the Naked Date. It's not an overnight sensation of choosing to do it, and then instantaneously being able to stand up against resistance. We have to *learn*.

The good news is, we *can* learn. And as we learn, we find the gifts of what regular intimacy brings to our marriage: love, ease, joy, humor, fun, delight, and, most importantly, pleasure.

When we have a regular time set aside for love, we start to relax with each other about being sensual and sexual. We stop worrying if our partner wants us enough to overcome the life pressures that usually stand in the way of intimacy and closeness. We know—no matter how the week goes—that we will be close or sexual, and so we ease up about the whole experience.

I believe, very strongly, that creating the habit of being intimate with our partner is a habit worth working on and worth having.

Maybe you've heard of Pavlov's dogs. Ivan Pavlov was a scientist who trained dogs to salivate at the sound of a bell. He used a bell to sound at a time when the animals would be fed, and when they heard the bell, their glands would secrete saliva, so that even when there was no food in front of them, their glands would still become active with the sound of the bell. That's what we're after with the Naked Date. To train ourselves to awaken our desire at the sound of the bell—at the appointed Naked Date time.

Does that sound regimented? Yes, of course it does! Particularly if we're still clinging to the myth of spontaneity. At first it seems that way, until we actually try it. The thing is, training ourselves to be open to sensuality at a particular time turns out to be relatively simple to do—and it works. The whole week can come crashing down on our head, but once we're in the groove of the Naked Date, our body, mind, and spirit will wake up to sensuality at the appointed hour. Sure, it takes a bit of time to get in the habit, but if we practice it for even a little while, we will start to get the hang of it. That's what we want: a regular expression of love, sexual connection, and intimate communion.

Sex and Science

If nothing else, a regular affectionate and sensual connection with our partner takes our stress level down a notch or two—a fact proven by dozens of scientific studies. Holding each other for even several seconds lowers blood pressure and creates easier breathing patterns, among other benefits. In a study led by Carnegie Mellon psychologist Sheldon Cohen that was published in *Psychological Science*, the researcher noted that hugging is a primary component of reducing the health risks of stress, the propensity for illness, and can even help reduce symptoms of people infected with colds. (http://reset.me/study/study-hugging-can-help-combat-stress-and-boost-your-immune-system/)

Also noted in the article, researchers at the University of Vienna found that oxytocin—the hormone released when we hold each other—reduces blood pressure, lowers anxiety, improves memory, and acts as a stress reliever. But it is not just hugging or holding once in a while that offers these affects. We must engage in them *regularly* to experience their benefits.

In the end, we're certainly after much more than just a stress reliever or combating anxiety. We're after a steady and sensual connection with our partner that makes us feel loved and adored, cherished and held dear.

Why should we care if we're "trained" to express love at a specific time? Because married life is not spontaneous. Couple for couple, the partners who have a Naked Date will connect intimately more often and more regularly *every time* compared to couples who don't have one. Regularity means consistent closeness, which makes us feel consistently loved. It relaxes us not only with its stress-relieving benefits, but also with its ability to help us experience trust and closeness.

We have to learn how to love well over time in order to make our marriage thrive. That means we need regularity in our loving acts. Big gaps in intimacy just won't work to promote passion, sweetness, and ease in our marriage.

We were never meant to be roommates in marriage. The truth is, the thing that distinguishes us from being roommates or best friends is intimacy. When we stop being intimate regularly, we start becoming distant. And we don't want that.

It's called "making love" for a reason

Intimacy is called "making love" for a reason. In sex, we are literally *making new love with each other.* We are creating a new bond—a deeper one, layered on top of the foundation we've already built—every time we engage in sexual intimacy.

Coming close shaves off the edges off our differences, and it cements us to each other. We can talk about it as a certain kind of magic, or we can speak about it metaphysically or scientifically, but it all adds up to the same thing: there is a lovely and mysteriously bonding thing that happens when we are satisfyingly intimate.

First, we let go. We stop holding on to little, petty irritations and focus on the good of our partner's heart. We notice the lovely things about him or her. We feel and act sweeter to each other. We may even go so far as to say that we are blessed by our partner's ability to please us. That the release, the ease, the heat, and the contentment that comes from making love together is a gift given, and so we hold it dear.

Sex takes the edge off. And though we're not looking to have only an acrobatic, press-for-a-release approach to making love—we want more than that—there is something to be said for a good, hot romp. It gives us a break from everything else—even if it's just for a half hour—and lets us set our brain on the shelf, so we can float in the land of delight and ease. That's not only good for the body, it's good for the heart and soul. And it's especially good for our marriage.

One of my girlfriends likes to say that when her husband has pleased her well she's less edgy about everything. "You go ahead and leave those socks *anywhere you damn please, babe . . .*" she'll say to him after a particularly good romp. And as humorous as that is, it's a truism. We are less edgy in our relationship when we are sexual with each other.

Sensuality is meant to be regularly woven into our experience of being a partner because it keeps us close. This is where the Naked Date can really help. Instead of worrying about whether our partner wants us enough to get his or her energy up for a sexual encounter, we know that we'll have one. Instead of pretending that it's fine that we're not making love, and that we "understand" that our spouse has had a hard week—while privately, inside our heart, we're rattled by our partner's lack of desire for us—we know that we will connect. It's already in the plan. We know there will time for lovemaking— holding, kissing, getting hot, getting sexual, and letting go into each other.

That tends to make us ease up. It helps us trust life a little more, and be more easy and gentle with ourself, and our partner. We field everything that our week throws at us better, and we tend to give our spouse some breathing room, too.

That's not to say that as long we have a bit of sex in our marriage that we should overlook a workaholic partner, a marriage-damaging habit, or some other tank-the-marriage issue. We need balance. That's what we're doing with the Naked Date. We are learning to map out some time for ourselves as a couple, to claim the good that's between us, and then own it and experience it. To *have* each other in the best sense of the phrase.

Sure, there are things that will come up to rock our steady Naked Date. Our partner might get sick. One person might break their arm or need surgery. One of us might be out of town for an extended time. A friend may show up from Spain and only have one night—Naked Date night—to visit. Things will come up over the course of a year; that's the way life works.

But when we have an ethic of getting to our lovemaking and connecting with our partner intimately, and we have a *strategy* to get to it regularly, we're ten times more likely to stay sensually connected than if we didn't. When we're sensually connected we're twenty times more likely to feel happy and well loved. And that's like striking gold in a marriage.

Making the time slot work in the real world

As a married couple, we need something that can help us check out together from life's demands. When we're twenty-four, that might mean a shot of tequila, a dance floor, and a bed. When we're older and more settled in our lives, we need a regular cue to help us get sensual on a consistent basis.

But just because we agree that the Naked Date is a good idea, and that we're willing to try it, doesn't mean we're going to master this right out of the gate. We're going to have to try it, work with the time slot, and if it falls flat, get back up and try it again a little differently.

We're going to have to see if Friday nights at eight actually *do* work. If they don't, maybe we'll need to try Saturday afternoon at three, when our teenage kids are gone so we can reasonably shut the bed-room door and get some privacy. We have to assess if the hour of the day is ticking our clock. We need to try it for a while and get back to each other on how our date time is panning out.

Are you too tired at your set time? Should you schedule an earlier time? Maybe weeknights are better than weekends because there are fewer kid or family events. Do you have small children? Maybe you need to impose a strict bedtime, rather than letting TV-time unravel into the evening hours that you could be using for intimacy. Maybe Sunday mornings at seven—even though that doesn't feel like it would be the sexiest time—is actually the time when you both have the most energy. Maybe you feel most refreshed on Saturdays at 10 a.m.

Know that no matter what, it's going to take about two months to perfect your Naked Date, so don't get frustrated if your early attempts don't work out on the first few times. Just keep trying it and varying it until the time you set starts to kick in the door on your resistance.

Don't choose a time that you know will be interrupted regularly. If you know your extended family always gets together on Sunday evenings every month or two, then that's not your time. If your kids often have birthday parties on Saturday mornings, then that's not your time. The Naked Date can be anytime you like, that's true, but it needs to be a regular weekly experience for the benefits to be felt in your marriage.

When my husband and I first did this, we figured out that we could reasonably address family events and social occasions on Saturday and Sunday evenings, so we made Friday our day. Now our friends and family know that we don't get together on Friday nights. If there's a pressing event scheduled on our evening, we only let those things break our date once or twice a year, at the most.

Lastly, know that at first you're going to be resistant to setting a time of day for your Naked Date. Your husband may *love* having intimate time in the morning, but somehow it just doesn't move you. Or your wife may love a late-night rendezvous, but late nights just leave you too exhausted. Know this: there will *never* be a perfect time that you'll both agree leaves you rested, totally present, and perfectly aligned with your life and desire cycles. You just have to choose the best time you can come up with, and then show up on a regular basis to be there for yourself and your partner.

Be of service in love

In my own marriage I have had to show up many a Friday evening when the world had just beaten me down, or when I was completely worn out from working and then fielding life's little disasters.

I've watched my husband do the same for me. To show up even though he's tired, worried, or exhausted, and then to put those emotions and feelings aside and give himself to me sensually, lets me know that he truly loves me. He's willing to give to me *even when it costs him something.* And that's heartening to me. It means I'm worth it to him. It means I'm important enough for him to make the effort.

The same is true for me. When I give, even when I'm not initially in the mood, I'm honoring him. I'm allowing him to arouse me, even when I feel tired or stressed, because it's good for me, good for him, and good for us. When I allow and permit that kind of willingness in our arousing experience, I always end up getting carried over the mountain of my resistance to thrill and grace and a terrific sexual experience. By showing up anyway and getting naked with him at our regular hour, I'm allowing for the possibility that my husband can lead me to love, and vice versa. And, it works.

That speaks to something else in our American approach to loving that we're not schooled in. We think we're always supposed to be in the mood. And, guess what? We're not always. That's just the way married life is. Many, many times—particularly before we get the hang of the Naked Date and our body begins to cue us—we will not feel like it.

But if we love our partner, and our partner has any physical expertise with our body at all, we can be drawn into a loving mood, *even when we think we can't.* That's the magic of the body. It's something I always talk about when teaching yoga: that we want to take our attention into our body and our breath, because the body has its own intelligence. It knows things. We have such an ethic of defining ourselves by our brain and the workings of our mind that's it often hard for us to find our sensual center. We need a sensual cue to remind us to put our brain on the shelf—its work is done for the day—and draw our attention down into the intelligence of our senses.

Put another way, we can learn to be of service to our marriage by showing up each week for our Naked Date. We have an opportunity to open up and offer ourself to love for the sake of ourself, our partner, and our marriage. That's the point of setting a time.

To show up for each other is an act of passionate commitment. We may do it as an act of love for our partner and our marriage at first, for sure, but later, as we practice it, our date time begins to carry us over into a mood-setting release, even when we think we weren't up for it. That's the power of this thing.

When we become willing to give, willing to receive, and willing to discover something new about how to practice our love and sex life, that willingness becomes the practical and physical road to a forever love affair. It's regular. It's true. It's sexual. And it deepens and lasts for years.

We build character by showing up for our marriage

There are three aspects of a relationship that need to be attended to: my being and needs, my spouse's needs, and the marriage's needs. The marriage is an entity all by itself, and just like a child or a creative project, we have to feed it and nurture it. So sometimes we have to show up for it when we don't initially feel like it.

Some Friday when I'm feeling, "Oh God, I'm so ridiculously tired and I just want to drop down on the floor and pass out from exhaustion," I say a little one-sentence mantra to myself that goes like this:

help me be of service to my marriage. And I let that carry me. Because my husband does have expertise with my body and knows the little tricks and sensual pleasures that draw me out and arouse me, all I really have to do is get next to him. When I do that—when I'm willing—I'm always pleased that we got naked, that I had sex with him, and we got close. I'm always better off when I overcome my resistance and make the effort to show up for the delight he offers me. And the same is true for him.

That regular practice of showing up for our marriage will, over time, build character in our marriages. Meaning, when we honor each other week in and week out, showing up for our appointed time together, our partner knows that he or she is worth the effort, and that will deepen our experience and our trust with one another, both sexually and in the marriage overall. Over time, our Naked Date will offer us an intimate trust that grows, as well as an openness with each other's bodies.

We absolutely want that. When we have that kind of willingness in our marriage, we blossom and bloom together. We literally let go into an experience of sensuality that carries us *someplace we didn't think we could go.* And that, my friends, is the whole point of a deepening intimacy.

"Bitchy" Wears Down the Intimate Soul

We all know couples who are always at each other. At every turn they cut the other person down, dismiss him or her, or get exasperated at some stupid little thing that should be a no-brainer to let pass by. They're *bitchy* with each other, and being around them is like being a lobster in a pot: the water just keeps getting hotter and hotter, and by the time you're done visiting, you feel like your skin is singed by their nastiness.

I'm not talking about bantering. Some couples love to banter: they love barbs and little ping-pong matches of verbal wordplay and some spicy belligerence in their daily talk. I'm not one of those people, and neither is my husband. In our marriage, we both have a terrific sense of humor about our foibles and regularly tease each other in good humor. But we don't like to verbally sword fight with each other just to get a rise out of the other person. But some people do.

My mother-in-law is ninety-five, and up until a few years ago, she had a seven-year relationship with a man who was two years younger, and they loved to bicker. One day I said to her, "You like a little piss and vinegar in your love affairs, don't you?" (She had that same sensibility with her late husband, too.) She smiled a knowing little smile at me and said: "Yes, I do, now that you mention it!"

All of that is fine as long as it's based on an underscoring of respect, kindness, soul-ease, and good will. And theirs was.

But it isn't always. A couple in our extended circle of friends constantly exuded a low-level—and sometimes visceral—anger towards each other for years. We knew he had a condition that rendered him unable to have intercourse, and that there had been no sex between them for years. And it showed. They were angry with their lot. Yet they hadn't done the things they could do to help themselves. And it just kept getting worse. She drank too much at parties and said nasty things to her husband and to other people. He was mean-spirited towards her and made snippy remarks. I used to look at them from across the room and wonder what had gone wrong. Even with a disability, the man's other faculties still worked; there were dozens of options for intimacy. All it would have taken was a little willingness.

That "disability" mentality is something we can all slide into. That somehow we're "blocked" from reaching our partner for one reason or another, and then we begin to have a kind of stand-off with each other, almost daring the other person to break through the ice cave we've surrounded ourself with. That meanness and pissy behavior is a taunt, and it's a time bomb. It's like saying, "You say you love me. Let's see you love me through *this*!" It's not the least bit honest or real or truthful. It's the worst kind of dare. *I dare you to take me on! I dare you to leave me! I dare you to talk about the elephant in the room because I damn well won't!*

Bitchy wears down the intimate soul. It kills desire. It's mean, and it's small, and it's totally and completely unnecessary. I'm not saying that we don't get angry and irritable and testy with our partner from time to time. We all do. But we can't live in that edgy, mean place—pissed that we're not finding the intimacy we really want, and turning our marriage into an icy standoff or a war zone.

If love is the answer, then sex and romance is the glue. When it breaks down, the whole rest of our relationship begins to disintegrate. And God knows we don't want that. It's awful. We get angry and rebellious and even mean-spirited when that happens. We're all going to have differences in our marriage, and sometimes we'll just have to agree to disagree—that's just life living with another human being. And we have to find ways to communicate about the big things in our life—kids, money, time, and how to make life choices. But we need to be able to do that with kindness, or we're never going to have a regular sex life together.

It is our romance and sensual intimacy that's going to keep us from getting so edgy that our differences take up all of the air in the room. It's the very heart of what will keep us connected and working on things together, willing to make our life together better and sweeter, no matter what comes up.

So we cannot—repeat *cannot*—ignore it.

The gifts of exploration

I once read a Chinese text that explained loving over the course of years. The idea was that a marriage, over time, was supposed to deepen sexually, not drift into canyons of separateness. The thought was that prowess developed with each other's bodies—through regular practice—would make us so close to each other that we could never imagine another lover touching us anywhere near as well as our partner.

Put another way, the more *time-in* we have with each other sexually, the more our prowess can grow and our love can deepen.

The belief was the exact opposite of our cultural stereotype about long-term love dwindling over time. In the Chinese text, more is better because—and here's the heart of it—by giving each other more and more sensual time over the course of years, we are offering the gifts of exploration and expertise to each other.

It's exploration in intimacy that will bring prowess, and that's exactly what the Naked Date offers us.

Uninterrupted time together

When we talk about prowess and time-in together, it begs the question: *how do we get that prowess?*

We get it by having *uninterrupted blocks of set-aside sensual time together,* and by building on those experiences week after week, month after month, and year after year.

Exploration in intimacy is much like exploration in artistry. Creative exploration requires quiet, contemplative time to nurture our ideas, and it also requires active, set-aside time where we can get our hands on our creative work to discover and practice what we have to say. It's unlike anything else in our goal-driven, linear, respond-to-this-notification timeline. Creativity asks us to work in the *nonlinear arena* of not knowing yet what we will create. It's a process experience, not a response-to-stimulus experience. It's freer, more amoeba-like, more open-ended. So we have to honor that need by giving ourself blocks of time that are given over to exploration.

When we show up for our creative or intimate time regularly, our inspiration tends to find us, without any hesitation. The writer Somerset Maugham has been quoted as saying, "I write only when inspiration strikes. Fortunately, it strikes every morning at nine o'clock sharp." That's exactly the theme we're playing out with the Naked

Date: we're setting aside uninterrupted, regularly scheduled time to let our sensual and sexual inspiration strike.

It's freeing to explore with our partner; to not know what we might find; to show up each week knowing *some* things about him or her intimately, but also to discover that *we do not know everything*. There is more to find out, there is more to experience. Engaging in that kind of exploration brings us prowess with our partner. It builds trust not only in our hearts, but also in our bodies. We're open to each other physically when we build a regular physical, sexual, and spiritual connection.

The way we get the gifts of prowess and bodily, sexual openness is to give our marriage steady and true blocks of time, without interruption, to explore our sensual life together. That's exactly what the Naked Date helps us do.

Jessica and Toby

Jessica and Toby had been married for more than fifteen years when we first spoke, and their sex life was, as Toby put it, "in the shitter."

Married in their early thirties, they had a steady and exciting sexual experience in the beginning. Over time, the pressures of two kids, jobs, her father's illness, and the buying up of local real estate in a quest to someday retire on passive income had taken its toll. Now they were now angry at each other, and their sex life had largely stopped altogether.

"I feel like he's not even here with me, even when we're in the house together. I have to tell him all the time to pay attention to things that need to get done. It's like he's sleepwalking when he's home, and it drives me crazy," Jessica explained.

Toby said, "I can't do anything right. Like the other night, she asked me four times if I fed the dogs. I mean, c'mon! How many times can I say, 'Yeah, I did it,' without getting pissed off?"

Seeing them together though, it was clear they really loved each other—and *liked* each other. They laughed quickly and easily at each other's jokes and had planned a huge anniversary event for themselves to renew their vows. So it was obvious they were not so distanced or angry that a few naked strategies couldn't help.

When we talked about which of the Naked Marriage strategies appealed to them, Jessica said, "We need help getting back in the sack. We're out there on separate islands, and we need to merge."

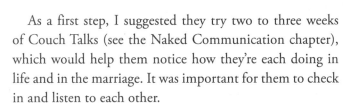

As a first step, I suggested they try two to three weeks of Couch Talks (see the Naked Communication chapter), which would help them notice how they're each doing in life and in the marriage. It was important for them to check in and listen to each other.

Several weeks later, when we met again, Jessica said, "This is going to sound stupid, but I didn't know half of the stuff that was going on in Toby's head—what he's worrying about or what's making him happy. Just talking is helping me get it."

Toby shared a similar sentiment: "I didn't realize that when I'm spacing out on her—trying to zero out on trouble, really—that that makes her come at me even stronger. She's trying to connect with me any way she can."

Next, I invited them to try the Naked Date. They set their time for Saturday mornings at seven. Since they're both early risers, and their preteen kids never get up before ten on Saturdays (and their bedrooms are well out of earshot), this was a reasonable time slot for them.

But they had to address getting in the mood. They came up with this strategy: they'd get up, brush their teeth and clean up a bit, and then make the bed, planning to be ready to be with each other by 7:15. Being intimate on a made bed, and then ripping back the covers at a particularly hot moment did something for them both.

Jessica had a thing about lingerie—it was a terrific sexual cue for her—so they incorporated that into their Naked Date. She'd put something on that was "for his eyes only" and let him watch her in it for a few minutes. When asked

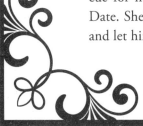

if this would work for him, Toby said, "Hell, yeah." She asked that he be completely naked—a turn-on for her as she watched him get aroused.

I advised them to go *very* slowly with their initial sexual touching. Given that there had been large gaps in their sensual exploration and connection, they'd want a steady, trust-building approach to their touch.

I also suggested some lifestyle changes. First, that they not add any property to their real estate "empire," and give themselves *one whole year* to just learn to enjoy each other again before adding anything to their plates. Second, I asked that they be as religious about their thirty-minute Couch Talks as their Naked Dates, recognizing that communication fuels intimacy. Third, I invited them to come to an agreement about who does what around the house, and to keep a chart if necessary, but then leave the other partner alone to do his or her "jobs" without commentary or criticism.

After a couple of months, they were having regular sex, they were talking regularly, and there was much more peace in their home life.

"It seems ridiculous to me that we needed a regular date to get next to each other sexually, but you know what? I don't care if it's ridiculous. It's working!" Toby said. "I love her so much more when we're talking and having some good sex."

Jessica said, "It still takes all of my willpower to keep my mouth shut about the way he's doing things around the house. But I get it. I was using that to punish him for not having sex with me. And now he is, and it's really good. We're laughing so much more, and we're listening to each other, and it's good for the first time in a very long time."

CHAPTER TWO
NAKED ROMANCE

What is romance?

Romance can be anything we want it to be. It could be becoming season ticket holders for the local women's basketball team. It could be taking a trek in the woods together. It could be building model trains together or planting tulips or cycling along the backroads of our hometown. All that matters is that we find something to do that lets us relax, and laugh together—something that gets us out of our regular, crazy routine so we can look at each other and have a little fun, and create some sensual glue.

Romance is important for one reason only: it gives us delighted access to each other's heart. Why do we want that? Because when we're in each other's heart we build desire. If we have no desire, we have no press to come back to each other and get naked. And we want that. It's good for us—good for our marriage, good for our partnership, good for our bodies and hearts.

Building sensual glue is what romance is all about. It's the stuff that will help us build upon and keep our Naked Date, and it's fun and delightful for its own sake as well.

We want to engage in things that bring us delight, joy, and lightness, because those things feel good and make our marriage a place of happiness.

There's another kind of romance as well: sexual romance. This is the stuff that gets our head into an erotic space, that helps cue our body and mind that it's time to make love. Each couple has these cues—ways we touch, present ourselves, look at one another, or reach for each other that says, *Mmmm, darling. I'm in the mood.*

But there's more to romance than just easy experiences and sensual cues. Every joyful, fun, sexy, and exploratory thing we choose to do together helps us build the regular intimacy that we're looking to experience and gives us more access to each other. It's a willingness to *play* we're talking about, which helps us build an easy, open road to intimacy.

Real love needs time to blossom

Most of us have been schooled in romance by popular culture—particularly by the tactile imagery of movies and television, which have worked into our imaginations the fast-action themes of what love is supposed to look like and supposed to be.

So let's take that apart for a moment. Filmic images are presented to us in distilled time—meaning that in order to propel a story in an hour-plus or a half-hour, the writers condense time, pick out the most dramatic parts of a story, and deliver it to us in a timeline that is faster than actual life. But, as with any theme that's fed to us over and over again, we tend to internalize the images of love instilled in us *the way they're presented.* Meaning, we often think the pace of love should be faster than it actually wants to be in "real life."

There are themes in the romantic images we're fed over and over again, for sure. These are:

1. Love is focused on twenty- and thirty-something people—those over forty are often presented as parents who are devoid of sexual energy, and not the focus of intimacy at all.

2. When sex occurs it happens right-quick, with no particular attention to foreplay or drawing out the passion of *both* partners, particularly the woman.

3. Finding love is a short, three-week "discovery" of passion, with barely a nod to the sensual life forged after the flash-and-dash union has been formed.

What I'm saying is that our images of love are often about "the chase," in a fast-action format, not about living in love over time.

We have tons of visuals showing ways to find new partners put in front of our eyes, with far fewer images presented of what it is to be *inside* a long-term love affair day to day. Particularly absent are images of sensual commitment over the course of years, in which a couple is portrayed as fulfilled in their romantic and sexual efforts.

The sexual revolution, for as much as it did to free us of stringent sexual mores, also did subsequent generations one grave disservice: it presented sex and intimacy as something we could drop in to, and slide back out of, quickly and easily, with the passion to "love the one you're with" as our guiding star. That gave some of us a skewed sense of what excitement is, meaning we attach sensual thrill to a new body, a new person, or a new experience. Mix that up in a cocktail with our images about youth-defined, fast and furious sexuality, and we have given ourselves only a tiny window of time for a shot-glass-down-the-throat experience of love, with no permission (in our imaginations) to sip, smell, and experience the taste of the sex-and-romance cocktail over the course of years.

We have a proclivity to think that finding a new and shiny partner is the only way to bring fiery passion and romance into our life, and that's a problem if we want to be in a devoted marital love affair.

We are unschooled at being successfully intimate in marriage over time. We defer to being busy instead of being romantic; we "forget" to engage in the sensual glue of having fun together, which sparks desire.

Real love needs time to blossom. Not only over the course of a marriage, but also over the course of sensual encounters. It needs attention to desire, a focus on arousal, and a drawing out of each partner on a regular basis. It requires *knowledge* of our partner's internal, sensual makeup. And that takes hours, days, months, and years.

As was mentioned before, in historical Chinese literature, it was thought that the "good stuff" in sex and love came only after years and years of a couple being together, when the man's prowess with his partner had gained an expertise that was unrivaled by any either could imagine, and a woman's ability to draw heat from her partner was unparalleled. It was based on experimentation, time-in with each other, and *mastery*.

It's the exact opposite of the messages with get from the images in popular culture today. Instead of a marriage dwindling in passion so that we become more like roommates, partners were encouraged to think of their sensuality as a long road of a deepening sexual prowess and expertise.

Sometimes, as Americans, we are an immature culture. We worship and idolize the wrong things. We miss the point of long-term love, thinking that it should be populated with the catch-fire, slam-and-jam exploration of bodies just discovering love for the first time. Sure, sex (and its power) is amazing in our teens and twenties, and it can be freeing and incredible, and even mind-bendingly ecstatic. But that kick-start flame isn't mature enough to last over the course of a marriage. It's only a beginning.

A great sensual marriage is a completely different animal than our first discovery of the sexual world. This animal is slower to arousal and needs time to separate itself from the duties of daily life long enough to find its sexuality and reconnect to it. It needs romance, fun, and ease.

It's a fire, for sure; when stoked and nurtured and attended to, it will burn slow and steady, fast and bright, or furiously and passionately, depending on the day. And that's its joy: it has levels and stages and discoveries and elations that crop up with different kinds of passions experienced over the course of years.

That's its gift—to experience it *all,* over time. So we've got to get inside it on a regular basis to get to the elation and the passion, as well as the steady and already-known stuff.

The upshot is, if we want a happy love affair, we need to put some hours into having some romance, too. The hour or two we set aside for sensual connection with the Naked Date needs that support to help keep our arousal accessible.

That means we want to *plan* for a bit of romance in our marriage, as well planning for our sexual time, and adapt ourselves to its nature.

The nature of romance is slow

When we talk about romance, we're talking about time set aside to draw each other out, to be with each other in a way that separates us from the workaday, checkbook-balancing, kid-juggling, crazy-scheduled world of our daily lives. I'd go even further than that: I'd call it holy, sacred, delight-inspiring time with each other.

To make something sacred is to separate it out from the mundane and the common, to approach it with a reverential humility. We need that kind of relationship to the time we set aside for our marriage's romance.

Romance—or, we might call it our sweet, joyous, and fun time with each other—doesn't come naturally in most lives. We often feel that we're too busy to take the time for recreational and romantic activities. More than that, when we do, we often need some ramping-down time from our overly scheduled lives to be able to focus on each other. That means the arc of using romance to stay connected is going to be *slow.*

Romance is the easy glue in our heart, the experiences that make us remember why we *like* our partner, which draws us closer when it's time to have sex.

Just like our reasoning for setting a Naked Date, life will never get still enough for us to have wide open afternoons for drifting into the garden together for a little poetry reading under a parasol. That's not our world anymore. And many of us wouldn't want that world. (We might crave something with a little more *juice,* a bit more edge and fire.) But whatever we want, if we want easy, romantic time together, we have to stand up for it, and then take it. It won't land in our laps without trying.

Remember that romance can be anything we choose. It doesn't have to be traditional romantic gestures. It could be a trek across the Pacific Trail, a Saturday morning breakfast date at your favorite café, a monthly gallery walk, or a nightly glass of wine in the living room while discussing the events of the day.

Romance is simply *anything that allows us to focus on each other one-on-one, enjoy each other's company, and see each other's loveliness.*

A reverential relationship to loving

To have a reverential relationship to our loving means we need a regular time to practice it. We can't casually expect that we'll just fall into the things that are truly important to us, and we wouldn't do that in any other arena of our life.

Think of anything else we do like a ritual: working out three times a week, taking a sculpting class, learning how to cook gourmet meals, going to a worship service, showing up for book club, becoming an experienced rock climber, playing in a Thursday night music circle. All of these things benefit from *practice.* They deepen in our hearts as a result of it. So, too, does our loving and romancing. That's the point here. If we keep treating romantic time as if it's an accidental occurrence that's supposed to spontaneously spring up from our psyches when "the time is right," then we'll never get any.

Of course, every couple has to determine what they want to share romantically. Traditional themes—flowers, candy, dinner—may not work, so we have to find the things that tick our partner's clock, and our own. That is the absolute key we're after: *what draws out our lover? What makes our partner warm to us?*

It's an art form to find that expertise in a marriage. To look and listen and try things, and see what works and what doesn't. To care enough to discover. To, over time, know that dressing up a bit and going out for a weekend cocktail will arouse your partner's ardor; that taking a walk hand-in-hand and just looking at the night sky will settle the two of you down and bring you close; that being naked in the bath together will do it for your partner every time.

We want the mastery of being able to *lead* our husband or wife into love. To stop thinking of passion as a hormonal experience for twenty-three-year-olds, and start living it for what it is: an adult, time-bound, mastery-seeking, exquisitely experiential ability to make our partner's heart and senses go from zero to one hundred, over an adult timeline, just because we led him or her there. Just because we *can*.

That's what romance is all about. Guiding and awakening, with the expertise of all of our sensual art forms, arousing our lover to love.

Kids, kids, and more kids

Before we start talking about the details of romance, and some ideas for it, we have to get practical about how to schedule a timeline for our romantic moments—and that includes our Naked Date, too.

Beyond the obligations of our outside-the-home world, many of us have kids, and we will have to negotiate our romantic time in relation to our parenting. So let's talk about the value of that.

One day I was at a gathering put together by a friend who was starting to give creative "getaway days" for women at her home. There were about ten women there, and I struck up a conversation with the woman next to me about romantic time in marriage. I said something along the lines of, "We've found that we need a weekly time to be alone and intimate with each other . . ." and the woman next to her—the mother of a four-year-old and an eight-year-old—rolled her eyes dramatically and said. "Yeah, right! Like that's going to happen. I'm a *mother*."

Her response knocked me back for a moment. Not because I'm unaware of the pressures of parents who have young kids—I'm not—but because as she continued to talk I realized she was taking this same stance with her husband. She was begging off from having intimate and romantic moments because she is a parent. That's not going to keep a marriage together.

Say all you want about the pressures of parenting—or the pressures of any of life's dramatic challenges—but if we use them as an excuse to not connect with our partner, we are going down a very bad road. Family life relies upon the glue between a wife and husband (or wife and wife, husband and husband in same-sex marriages.) When we start letting that glue get dry and crusty, it starts to chip away at the very foundation we're counting on for our family life.

Intimacy, plain and simple, is that glue. Going for months at a time without connecting with our partner sensually will, over time, take chunks out of the very bedrock we're counting on to keep our family intact. Our kids rely on us to keep our love and family together, so we have to have an ethic of doing just that.

Yeah, it's hard to get private time when our kids are young. We're exhausted, and there's a million things clamoring for our time and effort. But so what? Everything that's truly meaningful requires hard work, effort, and commitment. Why shouldn't our time together for pleasure—no matter how hard it is to make the timeline work—be on the top of our "to-do" list?"

That means we're going to have to train our kids to relinquish our attention long enough for us to have romantic time. On the flip side, we're going to have to take our attention *away* from them long enough to engage ourselves fully in our time with our partner.

When I was a small child, we had a gold area rug in the living room. My parents used to lie on the floor and hold each other, and then roll themselves up in the rug and kiss. My siblings and I would run around them, and laugh and tease them, yet they kept kissing. Then, every Saturday night they hired a babysitter, dressed up, and went to their favorite restaurant for dinner. They left us at home and went out to have some romantic time. Even when my brother was a baby and they had four kids under the age of seven, they continued this practice. They built into their daily life an expectation that there would be affection between them during our family time, and built into our psyches an expectation that they would have romantic time apart from us.

What I witness today—often among couples who had difficulty having kids and finally have them—is a reluctance to leave the children at home long enough to have some couple time. I had a girlfriend who bragged that she and her husband had never left their child alone once between her daughter's birth and her seventh birthday. Their child determined all of the time constraints, consumed all of the focus, and it was evident that the couple's focus on each other had faded and lapsed.

Then sometimes there's a kind of obsession with our children that pops up. I have some acquaintances who have a toddler—and God knows a toddler takes up a ton of attention—and one parent has an uber-focus on every move the kid makes that's full of worry and obsession. The non-obsessing partner is not allowed to help and ends up looking off into the distance as if there's no possible way to intervene. One partner is sidelining the other in favor of a hyper-attentive focus on the toddler, while the other is drifting, not speaking up for the marriage. This is not a balanced family experience, and it won't work for keeping the basis of our family—our love connection with our spouse—healthy. Our partnership is the primary bond. Not our kids. And as compelling as it is to turn our full attention to our new baby, our toddler, our young kids or our teens, if we leave our partner out in the cold, we will chip away at the very core of what holds our loving family together. We will, without doubt, put our family at risk.

We have to find balance. Though it's not always easy, with a little practice and a few simple shortcuts applied, we can realistically do it.

Love is an active verb. Love needs attention and practice and reverence to make it work. So we can't use our kids as an excuse to avoid loving our partner—not if we want the closeness we say we want; not if we want the passion we say is meaningful to us. We have to stand up, show up, and build a platform from which we can experience our loving over time. And then, and only then, can we claim the good of our intimacy, our marriage, and our whole family experience.

Making time in the real world

Most of us aren't resisting love on purpose, we just get bowled over with all of the things in life that distract from it. So what do we do if we have babies or small children and we really want to institute some sensual and romantic time in our week? How do we manage that?

If we've got small kids, we need to think about how much time we need and plan for it. Sexually, we probably need at least one undisturbed hour per week to be with each other. But sensually, we may need more. We may need and enjoy a bit of ramp-up time to reconnect from the week, to see each other outside the lens of daily life, and to view each other the way we would on a date. In other words, we may need a little time to get in the mood.

As I said before, I'm not looking to tell anyone how to manage their romantic life. You're going to have to set that up with your partner, based on what you both need and want. But what I do know is this: a regular, weekly, set-aside-for-intimacy date with each other keeps our marriages fresh and loving and true to each other, and *at least one hour* of doing something pleasurable together, no matter how simple, fuels our romance and kick-starts our desire. It binds us and bonds us in the sweetest of ways.

Even when it feels like an extreme effort to make it happen, it is worth every ounce of that effort.

Genevieve and Carey

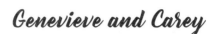

Carey and Genevieve met in high school. They were the "it" couple—she was a band majorette, and he was a star basketball player—and dated for the full four years.

When they went away to college, they both planned to return to their small hometown after graduation and kept up a long-distance love affair.

"That was the sexiest part of our relationship," Genevieve stated. "It was day-in and day-out longing for each other. We ran up huge phone bills!"

"I hated busses, and I took the bus six hours twice a month to see her," Carey said.

"We had these steamy weekends, and we wandered around my college town doing nothing, just holding hands and hanging out. It was so good," Genevieve explained.

After twenty years of marriage, living in the small town they grew up in, they both admitted that their romantic life has "largely disintegrated," as Carey put it. "There's no place to go where we don't know everyone, even in the neighboring towns—we've been here so long. Friday night at our favorite fish hangout or the pizza place turns into a high school reunion, and there's no time that's just ours."

"I guess that's my fault," Genevieve added. "I'm a talker and everyone knows it. Since I work at city hall, everyone comes up to me to find out what's going on."

They have three kids who are involved school sports, so much of their time is spent driving to and sitting through games, which they enjoy, but, as Genevieve noted, "It's family time, not our time."

When I asked how the lack of romantic, one-on-one, focused fun time was affecting their marriage, Carey piped up first. "I don't know about her, but I just feel like it's business as usual. Nothing for me, nothing for her, nothing for *us*. And that bums me out."

Genevieve had no idea what Carey was feeling. "I figured this is our life right now, until Carey told me he wasn't happy. It was like a knife through my heart. I thought we were okay," she said.

When asked about their sex life, Genevieve asked, "Does it have to be about sex? Why can't it be about companionship?" I like having sex with him—being 'intimate' as you say. But just because we don't do it a lot of the time doesn't mean I want to lose him."

They both agreed that adding some one-on-one romance or fun time might help them bring some vibrancy to their intimate life. I suggested they begin simply without a lot of pressure to perform—to just agree to find ways to hang out together.

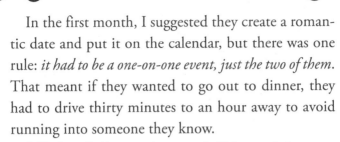

In the first month, I suggested they create a romantic date and put it on the calendar, but there was one rule: *it had to be a one-on-one event, just the two of them.* That meant if they wanted to go out to dinner, they had to drive thirty minutes to an hour away to avoid running into someone they know.

"I'll drive!" Carey volunteered. "It's worth it to me to get some alone time with you." They agreed to take not only a night, but an afternoon and an evening in another town each Saturday.

Since their kids were older, they didn't have to hire a babysitter, but they did have the challenge of training their kids that they wouldn't be parentally available on Saturdays. They might miss a game or two and sometimes had to entrust dropping off and picking up the younger kids to their seventeen-year-old daughter, but they agreed it could work.

Carey started mapping little towns to discover within sixty to ninety minutes from home. On Saturdays they'd take off at around noon for one of their "journeys," as Genevieve called them.

Since they didn't have tons of money to throw around, Carey researched to find places to eat that were affordable and still nice enough to feel romantic. I suggested they try what my husband and I do: hit some happy hours with inexpensive food in nice restaurants.

If they were totally out of cash at the end of the month, then they agreed to put together a picnic with a bottle wine and find a town center or park to eat in.

"I felt this idea was high maintenance at best," Genevieve admitted to me after a couple of months. "But I agreed to try—to be *willing* for the sake of my marriage, as you like to say, so I went along with it. Now I'm feeling the way I did when we were in love in college and we'd have those romantic weekends after being apart. We're just wandering around holding hands and looking at things, being together. It's easy."

After a month, I invited them to apply the Naked Date—to choose their time, lock their bedroom door, and let the kids know they needed privacy. Their romantic time made them feel good about hanging out together again, and exploring helped them become willing to play a little bit more, which helped their sex life.

"I'm loving this," Genevieve said. "We got so kid-focused and work-focused that we forgot about *us.*"

"We're actually laughing in bed," Carey added. "It's happiness laughing. We're *tickled* with each other again. I don't know how that happened, but it's happening."

Romance comes in two parts

Romantic time, by my definition, is a two-part process. There's the romance of easy, fun, light-hearted experiences with each other, and then there's the before-sensuality romance that fuels the sensual hour or two of our Naked Date.

When my husband and I first started showing up for our Naked Date, we were keyed into having some intimate time in bed. As we began to progress with the thing, and we began to trust that we would actually get naked and be intimate each week, we realized there were some romantic cues we could use that would allow us to deepen the experience.

For us it was pretty clear: we love to dress up a bit and go have a drink or an appetizer out. Our spending parameters don't allow us to go out for a swanky meal every week—and we don't want to be stuffed with food when we're having sex anyway—but we can put aside enough money to hit our favorite restaurant happy hour, to sit and feel elegant and separate ourselves from our workday personalities for an hour or so before we engage in our naked intimacy. We can look at each other, chat a bit, have a little something to eat, and then head home for a good romp.

That feels like romance to us—a nice, slow, ramp-up for our sex time together.

We also do other romantic things, separate from our Naked Date. We go to a film together, and then stop by our favorite East Indian café. We take a walk in our neighborhood. We lie on the bed while my husband reads something out loud. We go up to the reservoir trail near our flat and hike for an hour or two. All of these things allow us to *focus on each other,* which is what we're after.

For you it may be something else. And you'll have to find those things for your marriage: the things that help you both open up to sensuality when it's your set naked time, and the things out in the world that help you relax together and focus on each other.

One thing I can tell you about romance: it's *not* flopping down in front of the television and expecting your partner to come and sex you up. It's not obsessively busying yourself in the kitchen, waiting for your husband or wife to come and break the adrenaline-cycling of your cleaning and tidying. It's not letting your kids consume every bit of your couple time, letting them watch TV every night until late in the evening, and then expecting your partner to generate sensual feelings for you at eleven o'clock at night out of thin air.

The key to romance is this: *focusing on one another while having a pleasurable experience.*

Romantic and intimate time that's right for you

I was at a dinner party and started talking about the Naked Date. One woman, the mother of two small kids, said, "That's such a great idea! Saturday night at ten is perfect for us!" When I asked her if she thought they'd both have energy at that hour, she said, "Absolutely. We're both always up until midnight." With the kids in bed, the TV turned off, and a little zeroing in on each other sensually, they were able to institute a bit of living room romantic time that led them right into their Naked Date. And they did it without having to leave their house.

Romance is about paying attention to each other, and doing just what this couple did: finding a way to focus on each other so they could move toward each other easily.

That means our support systems need to aid that process. If being at home zaps our energy or distracts us from love, then we need some time away from home to connect with each other. If it doesn't and we can find romance at home, then that's terrific!

For many of us who have kids, though, in order to get that romantic time we need to remember these three magic words: *get a babysitter.*

What to do if you can't afford a babysitter

If we want a regular loving experience, and our focus on kids (or even dependent relatives) is not allowing for it, then we need a support system so that we may claim and experience the loving hours we need. We need *regular coverage each week* so we can get to our intimacy and romance.

But what if we can't afford a sitter?

Most of us are not rolling in cash, so when I casually say, "Hey, get a babysitter for three hours every weekend," I know I'm asking you to do something that comes at a price. But there are creative ways to approach this that can get you the romantic time you need at a fraction of the cost.

First, being thoughtful about romantic time—planning for it—means we have to plan for it financially, too. It has to be a priority. As I said in my last book *How to Be an Artist*, if we're not willing to learn how to set aside time for the things we say we want, it's like continuing to put scraps in the compost bin and expecting it to smell sweet. We're in for a rude and decomposing awakening if we think we can find love and happiness with no effort.

So we have to make our money plan dovetail with our priority to have a romantic experience on a regular, weekly basis. Do we need to break the bank to have a little time out together? No. I'm saying that with a little thoughtful *clarity* we can plan for what we need in proportion to our income. (We'll talk about how to do this specifically, point-by-point, in the *Naked Money* chapter.)

Let's say your family is totally crunched for cash—maybe one of you is out of work—and since you're stressed, you both recognize the need to get away from home-based family responsibilities and money concerns to keep your loving bond strong. What can you do?

The simplest thing to do is to make an arrangement with another couple to trade nights of babysitting. Lots of our friends who have small kids use this method, even if they're not pressed for cash. Our friends Keyla and Evan have great neighbors, and on Friday nights they leave their daughter with them for three hours. Then, on Saturday night, they take the neighbor's child. And it works out terrifically. That said, things come up, so they do have a sitter in the wings in case there's a conflict one weekend. So they set aside a little cash to cover that expense.

Another couple we know has pre-teens. Their two boys do the neighbor's yard work and mow the lawn every week, and then that couple takes the boys for a couple of hours each Sunday night. The parents give the boys a little allowance for doing the neighbor's gardening, and everybody's happy.

Other couples I've coached have family members—grandparents in particular, or aunts and uncles—who they can ask to sit for them. It doesn't really matter who you choose, you just want to make it work so that you get some romantic and sensual time. You may want the sitter to come and stay with the kids, or you may want to drop them off at the sitter's so you can be at home alone for your sensual time. Or you may want to go out first—even for a walk. It doesn't matter what you choose to do, it just matters that you take the time due to you as a loving couple.

Don't choose people in your circle who use you for the sitting service and then cancel on you when it's your turn. (If that happens twice without advance and equal notice, get rid of them and find someone else.) Don't choose family members who are nosy and judgmental about the two of you taking time to be together romantically, and, in particular, stay away from jabbing-and-cutting parents who tend to tell you that you're selfish for wanting time alone. Step back from any relatives who may try to nose in on what you're doing every week, or family members or friends who make snide comments about your efforts to stay connected in your marriage.

In other words, though your sitters don't need to know the details of your Naked Romance or Naked Date commitments, stay away from people who will sniff it out and try to make you feel bad about it. There are always people who will try to make you feel bad for doing a good thing for yourself and your marriage. Stay far, far away from those people. Go where the love is. Go where there is understanding and kindness. Set up your foundation for romantic time with that ethic, and then unapologetically *take the time* you set aside for romance, love, and sensuality.

Remember that no one's going to arrange this for you. So set it up, support it, claim it, and then own it. If you want love, you've got to stand up for it and take it.

Sex and romance—with teenagers in the house

Teenagers present a wholly different challenge to romance and sex between partners. First off, teenagers are coming into their own sexual awakenings, and their biology has them noticing every little wisp of eroticism the wind blows in their direction.

So it's best, in my opinion, to be honest about what you're up to, particularly if you're going to try to take your intimate time when they're in the house. That doesn't mean you have to tell them the blow-by-blow of what you're about to do. What we're after is the ability to go upstairs and *close the door,* no matter which child is at home, and have our privacy respected.

It's best, then, to have a conversation with them about the rules for when you're behind the closed door. Here's a suggestion of what you could say: "Your mother and I [or father and I] are going to start taking some intimate time together when we're home. Our marriage is the bond that keeps our whole family together, so we need some time alone with each other. When our door is closed, you're not allowed to interrupt unless it's a real emergency."

Because teenagers will sometimes take this as a challenge to test the boundaries, you've got to be specific about what an emergency is: someone is bleeding heavily; someone has been knocked out on the floor; the dog is choking and has stopped breathing; water is pouring from the upstairs bathroom onto the kitchen floor—these are emergencies. The television has bleeped out, the computer game has stalled, one sibling is pissed at another for stealing a football jersey out of the other's closet—these are *not* emergencies.

You must be clear that if they interrupt your closed-door time, there will be consequences. Their phone gets taken. They're grounded. The best thing to do when your privacy is not respected is to throw an elbow. When you hear the interrupting knock and the whiny complaint that one sibling is not letting the other use the remote, *just don't answer.* Don't say, "Go away," or "We told you not to . . ." Just don't respond. After a time or two, your teenager will get the message and go away. Whatever the interruption, when you *know* it's designed to test your limits and interrupt your naked time, it cannot be passed off as cute. It's not. It's disrespectful and a challenge to your ability to have an adult love life.

I'm not saying don't have a good laugh about it. It's funny how fast kids pick up on our sexual bond, particularly if we have not been taking time with each other before now, and they will—in some Freudian way—sometimes take it as a subconscious challenge. But as long as we set boundaries and don't bolt out of bed to try to settle a teenage argument, and we stand our ground, they'll get the message quickly enough.

Teenagers sometimes have activities on Friday or Saturday night, which can leave us alone at home from time to time, and when that happens it's nice to use that time for intimacy. But we can't wait for that. We need our intimate time to be regular. So if one child is a social butterfly and loves to go out with friends and the other is a couch potato, then we may have to institute closed-door time when they're at home.

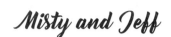

Misty and Jeff

"We're just not the romantic type," Misty noted the first time we spoke. "We're more the hang-out-in-gym-shorts-and-sweats kind of couple."

"We work all the time, and when we do see each other, we're with our kids—very verbal kids who need lots of attention," Jeff explained. "They wear us out."

The previous year, Misty took on a second job to help them save for a house, which all but ensured that they barely saw each other, and by the time she'd get home she could barely hold her head up.

"All she ever says to me these days is, 'I'm so tired.' It's like a song I hear every night, 'I'm-so-tired-I'm-so-tired,' and then she's conked out," Jeff said.

"I'm not liking this any more than he is," Misty added. "We get a little sex in once a month or so, and that's all we get of each other."

They were living in an expensive area and had modest incomes, so there wasn't cash to get a babysitter and go out for a nice dinner or get a hotel room just for fun—things they had done when they were first dating.

"I feel beaten down, that's the issue," Misty said. "My doctor says I'm headed for some kind of fatigue syndrome if I don't knock it off, but what can we do? We're trying to get ahead here."

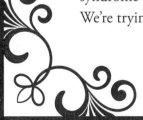

Their issues were bound up in two things: 1) the need to keep their marriage together for their own sake and the sake of their kids, and 2) the need to make lifestyle and money choices that would offer them a chance to do that.

I suggested two things right off the bat: first, since they had an extra vehicle, I asked if they'd be willing to sell it and put the money in an account for fun and romance, which would give them money for a babysitter, a meal out, or a movie *at least two times a month* for several years. Second, to make their date night work, Misty had to give up a shift at her second job (a restaurant) on Saturday nights.

She balked: "That's messing with my plans."

I asked her if having a house and money in the bank was worth it if she lost her health or her marriage.

"It's not okay with me that we have nothing for us, Misty. We have to do this," Jeff urged.

Misty agreed.

It took almost a month to get several babysitters lined up so they'd have a fallback and always get their time together. They booked their sitters weeks ahead and wrote their Naked Romance dates on the refrigerator calendar in red ink.

"I see that date coming up and I think, 'Thank God,'" Jeff said. "Just starting this has been a lifeboat for me."

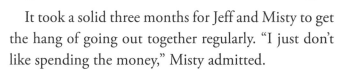

It took a solid three months for Jeff and Misty to get the hang of going out together regularly. "I just don't like spending the money," Misty admitted.

I started working with them on their spending (see chapter five), and as they began to get clarity with their finances, Misty began to relax about having some money set aside for them to have fun together as a couple.

"Until we started being clear about our money, I just wasn't okay about spending it on us," Misty said.

Understanding her concern, Jeff said, "I look for free events for her, too, especially now that we're going out every weekend. Concerts in the park, a free movie event. We even went to a trivia bee at the college here. I took her river rafting last month, and that was awesome. But the main thing is we're getting out together every week and having some fun. It's life-changing."

It took them a few months to try the Naked Date as part of their romance and intimacy efforts. That made sense, since they hadn't been spending enough time together previously to generate desire.

"It was just airplanes buzzing by the tower with us before," Jeff recalled. "Once we got a little one-on-one time, our sex life got better."

"We agreed to see what would happen naturally, and though it didn't get as regular as once a week, we

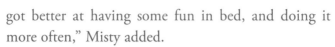

got better at having some fun in bed, and doing it more often," Misty added.

Then, Jeff decided he wanted to try having some naked time after their romance time, with no pressure to have sex. "We tried it and this magical thing happened: we scheduled being home from our time out at ten or ten thirty, and then we'd get right in bed and see what could happen. We started having fun doing that, and then one thing led to another."

"It's great," Misty said. "The kids are in bed, we've just had some fun, we're still awake, and we're both willing. So suddenly we've got this regular sex life again, and it's making us both happier and looser."

Several months later, they told me they were moving to a smaller town in another state. "A place where we can buy a house, raise our kids, and have time for a decent, loving marriage," Jeff said.

"He finally put his foot down," Misty explained. "One job apiece, a place we can relax and have a real marriage and a happy family. 'Our marriage has got to come first,' he told me. And he's right."

No trash talk allowed

There's one more piece of our romantic life that's important to address when we're negotiating our Naked Romance or Naked Date time with teenagers (or other relatives) in the house. We need to nip in the bud the trash talk they dish out when we're affectionate in front of them.

You know what I'm talking about. You come around the corner and see your wife dressed up to go to a party with you and you say, "Wow, hon. You look hotter than the first time I saw you." And your kid loudly says, "That's just so *gross!*" Or you spot your husband out the window working in the yard with his shirt off and you say out loud, "He looks gorgeous even when he's a sweaty mess." And your teenager quips, "That's *disgusting*, mom." Or the two of you pass each other in the hallway and stop and kiss and wrap your arms around each other, and your teen says, "Stop it! That's sickening."

You've got to cut those comments off at the pass. They will not help you feel entitled to your own adult sensual life, and they're not—by a longshot—helping your kids understand the nature of what a long-term, loving marriage needs to survive and thrive.

The thing I often say to teenagers when they start spouting that *parents-and-romance-ick* thing is this: "When you're old enough to be in a serious relationship, won't you want the person you marry to love you all your life? Won't you want them to hold you and kiss you and be intimate with you? Isn't that what *forever* means?"

Another way to express this is to take your teen aside and tell them that support, compliments, and being proud of them—for good grades and good games, for doing their homework, for looking good before the winter dance, and for just being a good person—is exactly what they want from you. Then tell them that just because someone becomes an adult doesn't mean the need for approval and affection goes away. The difference between being a good parent or a bad parent is that the good parent has an ability to make their child feel special in the world . . . and the same thing is true of being a good partner. These needs don't stop when we're thirty or forty or even eighty.

Our teenagers need to be taught this. So we need to let them know it's not okay to make cutting comments about the efforts we make to be a loving couple, especially when we're affectionate in front of them. Open affection is part of a fulfilling marital experience over time, and they need to learn this if their own marriages are to succeed.

One of the terrible things we do to our teenagers is we don't prepare them for how to be good partners in marriage. Maybe we teach them about preventing pregnancy and disease, and maybe, if we're kind, we let them know that the growth and expression of their sexuality is normal and natural. But what we don't do—as a whole culture of parents—is teach them how to love over time, sensually and deeply, in a marriage. So stepping up and being an example of what loving affection and appreciation looks like is truly one of the best things we can do for them.

We want them to learn that if they're lucky they'll meet someone in life who will treat them in the same cherished, adored, romantic, and desired way that we are treating our partner.

So don't let your children disparage your loving, or denigrate your appreciative or even flirty behavior. Don't allow that commentary in your house. If your son or daughter wants to talk privately to their friends about how *weird* it is that their parents are affectionate, then fine. But not out loud in your home.

We are the only close-up example our teenage kids are going to get for how to love over the course of years. So at the very least we can prepare them to think about what a loving marriage looks like by taking the time we need for love and affection, and by not allowing them to interrupt us, sideline us, or badmouth us for it.

Weaving an experience of ardor

Naked romance is the ramp-up to the Naked Date—it's the ease-into-it time that helps each of us separate ourselves from the slammed world of our daily life and helps us turn our attention to love. So whether it's a romantic or fun act engaged in just before our Naked Date, or an out-in-the-world event sometime in our week, we need to talk about what it looks like specifically so we can get to it.

To get to the heart of it, we can ask these simple questions: *What can I do, week in and week out, that will help quiet my partner's head and help draw him or her into the world of the body and the senses? What can I do to enter into open and attentive willingness to draw my partner into love, fun, and companionship? How can I warm my partner's heart to ardor?*

Ardor is a beautiful word. The dictionary defines it as "passion, fervor, enthusiasm, zeal, emotion compelling action; devotion, feelings that are deeply stirring or ungovernable."

What I love about this definition is what's in the middle of it: *emotion compelling action.* Meaning ardor is much more than just feeling something; it asks us to *act.* It asks us to find our want and our desire, and then do something about it. That's a perfect definition of what we're up to with the Naked Date, and what we want in our Naked Romance. We want our devotion and our love to be visible, to be tactile, and to be able to be felt by our partner. This is a good basis for thinking about what kind of romantic actions will work for our marriage.

If we want to weave an experience of ardor together, we're going to need experiences and cues that help us get there. We're going to need relaxing and connecting experiences, and sensual and sexual cues. And we will talk about each in turn.

But first, let's ask ourself this: what constitutes an amorous experience? What helps draw two partners into intimacy and closeness?

Offer each other relaxing, fun, connecting experiences.

The most important part of romance, as we said before, is this: *we must get away, by ourselves, and engage in something that allows us to focus on each other.* This is the starting point.

As we mentioned before, there are two categories of romance: 1) relaxing, fun experiences, and 2) amorous ones.

When we talk about finding relaxing and connecting experiences, what we really mean is doing things that we do exclusively together—that is, things we do outside the home, or inside it, to relax with each other one-on-one; things that bring a sense of shared, private intimacy. They are events or experiences that separate us from the daily work world, from our parenting responsibilities and family time, with their sweetness and their ability to let us focus on each other and find delight in each other.

For some couples, as it is for us, that's going to be dressing up a bit and going out for a cocktail or dinner. For others it might be sitting on the back porch, holding hands, listening to sixties music. Some couples may want to take an experiential class together, like painting or music appreciation or a travelogue class; some might want to learn how to make pasta together or join a wine tasting club. These are romantic things you'll do separate from your Naked Date—things you do one-on-one to relax together and have fun.

Though we want to be open to our partner's needs and our own, we want the activity to work for both of us. For instance, I'm always dying to take some dancing lessons with my husband, but when I bring it up he says, "Yeah, I'll go. But on one condition: I only want to dance with you. I have no interest in dancing with other people. If we do it, I want to do it for you and me." And I agree. The romance, for us, is in learning to dance together. So when we go looking, we have to find a class that allows us to do that.

When my father-in-law was still alive, he and my mother-in-law came up with a great compromise for their couple's activity. She loved everything to do with women, politics, and activism. He loved every sport on the planet. He suggested they become fans of the Stanford women's basketball team. They did, and both ended up loving it. Still today, years after his death and at the age of ninety-five, she gets season tickets and goes to every game. My husband and I know that the simple, relaxing act they engaged in together still lives on in her heart in a romantic way, so she still goes, has some fun, and remembers him.

We're looking for those kinds of activities—things we can do together that we both enjoy, and that help us relax and feel connected, things that bind us experientially. We're looking for *special*.

Television and movies really don't do the trick, sorry to say, because we don't focus on each other while we're watching them. They can be relaxing, sure, but they don't often leave us feeling romantic and close for one simple reason: we are each off in our own little world, with our faces focused on something besides our partner. As one of my girlfriends once said, "I sit there and I watch this cable show he loves, and it's full of manipulators and mind-benders and nasty people, and it's not even close to a romantic experience, but I want to be next to him, so I do it." That experience is fine to have, but it doesn't pass for romance.

Romance requires the ability to value each other's company—or at the very least, engage in a shared experiential event. So we've got to be more inventive than just plopping down in front of a screen and thinking that's going to work.

Traditional cues work for a reason

Then there are the traditional romantic cues: dinner, candles, candy, flowers, cards. They're cliché and classic for a reason: they work. They play on our hearts simply and easily because they are icons for us—we know what they mean. Sometimes we blow them off because we think they're too cliché, but we shouldn't. What's woven into these traditional acts of romance is *kindness* and *thoughtfulness*.

When my husband brings me a single rose in the middle of the day for no reason at all except that he loves me, it tells me that he has been thinking of me when he's away from me. When I find a loving card and write a note thanking him for all he gives to me, and hand it to him on a day that's not his birthday or a holiday, it lets him know that he walks with me in my heart when I'm out in the world without him.

These little gestures are heady and powerful messages for the heart. They are every bit about romance: we are thinking of the other person when we are out in the world, and we *long* for her or him. If we want lasting passion, we have to offer more than just jumping into bed and getting sexual. We have to practice *cherishing each other*. These traditional acts of romance work for that reason.

There's not one person on this planet who doesn't respond to being loved, being cherished and appreciated. Not one. That means we don't want to forget birthdays, anniversaries, or holidays. We want to make an effort to appreciate our partner on other days, too, when he or she is not expecting a card or flowers or a small gift. We want to engage in the romanticism of appreciation—the delicious juice that sweetens the cocktail of love and softens the heart.

If you're a woman, don't expect your partner to do all of the flower buying or to always initiate romantic outings. Yes, it's a strong aphrodisiac to have a man make the arrangements for a "date," to have him open the door for you and seat you in your chair. But buy him some flowers once in a while. Take some initiative, too. Plan something sweet for him, and take the lead on arranging from time to time.

For men, don't make your partner drag you kicking and screaming to an event together, or make her beg to get a small gift and a card during the year or on her birthday. Make an effort. Participate. Lead a little.

Partners respond to chivalry, to thought that has gone into making a nice event for both of you. Do it on your own terms and make it come from the heart, but do it. That's what the connective glue of ardor is all about.

Lead your partner to love. That, in a nutshell, is the definition of Naked Romance.

Sensual and sexual cues

The second category of romantic behavior includes the sensual cues we offer each other in the privacy of our own home or bedroom. Sometimes, when we look at our intimate life, we think we don't have any cues that can help our partner open up to sex or getting naked, or we don't see anything he or she is doing to cue us. Pay attention. Each marriage has its own cues, its own rituals for opening up to one another.

He might have a way of touching your ass that lets you know he's thinking sexual thoughts; she might have a way of stroking your inner thigh that let's you know she's open to sex play.

If you don't like the cues you have, then experiment until you find something that ticks your partner's clock, and your own.

In my own marriage, I know good and well that the only thing I ever have to do to arouse my partner's sensual interest is to put on a pair of high heels. He will, in a split second, drop whatever is in front of his face—the newspaper, his computer, a book, or a football game—and will spin his head toward me the *minute* he hears the click-click of my high heels on our wood floors.

He also has a terrific artistic eye, so me being half-naked or in some fun or provocative outfit that's crafted to be artistic will always turn his head and open him up to some intimacy. Since I love to dress up, and love to feel sexy in front of him, this is an easy romantic cue for us to play with. After years of being together, our cues have become ingrained in us, and a bit Pavlovian—we know what will work, and we use them as shortcuts to get into our loving without a lot of muss or fuss. By using them, we can come up behind each other at the kitchen sink, when the other is not remotely in the mood, and turn each other's attention to sex.

How did we discover this? The high heels thing has a special relationship to us in our marriage. I'm about the same height as my husband, so when I put on a pair of three-inch heels, I'm quite a bit taller than he is. At the beginning of falling in love with him, I asked him if he'd prefer that I wear flats. He said, "Absolutely not! I love you in high heels. It means we're different than everybody else, and I find that sexy." That's all it took. High heels became a private language of sexy and different for us—special, in other words—and we cued into it together and began to use this simple spin to enhance our sexual ramp-up.

Does that mean I always have to go to extreme fashion efforts to arouse him every time we're intimate? Does It mean I'm always teetering around in high heels? No. I use the cue when I'm in the mood, or he asks me if I'd like to put on some heels for him. It's a sign that one of us is interested, an offer of sex. It's also a terrific cue that I can use on our Naked Date night to help our erotic imaginations ease into our sexual sensing. Because we have it, we can use it to get sexed up. That helps us on the Fridays when we want to connect with each other, but need to overcome tiredness or resistance.

That's the point of a romantic cue. It works to draw us into a sensual place. Does it mean we're always going to have sex every time we play with that cue? No. It's sex play. It's light, and it's easy, and sometimes, say during the week, it leads to a full-blown romp, and sometimes it's just foreplay for another day. On our Naked Date days, it helps to get us ramped-up for the intimate, sexual loving we're committed to having each week.

It's a good idea for each partner to have a sensually romantic cue to offer the other. My husband has a ridiculously simple cue for me. I love to see him naked. It's that direct for me. I always feel like he's most beautiful without clothes—that his real beauty is hidden from the world, and that makes me feel like it's just mine. That's a powerful enough aphrodisiac for me. Does he have to be perfectly ripped for me to feel this way? No. He exercises and takes care of himself, but he's not perfect—none of us are. That's not the point. The point is to find something I adore about him, and for me it's the privacy of those moments when he can make me follow him into the bedroom just by getting naked for me. That's powerful.

Dancing is also a big cue for us. My husband will ask me to dance with him—naked or clothed—in the living room. That'll do it for me every time, too, and he knows it. He can use these sensually romantic acts to help draw me out of myself long enough to connect with him. That mastery—the prowess he has to draw me into love—is sexy for me all by itself. He moves me with it: by wanting me, by knowing what will work to draw me out. And that's the point.

Once again, it doesn't matter if our romantic sex play blossoms into full-blown sex each time. In fact, it's fabulous to have little dips into the ice cream carton of love without having a whole bowl. (We'll talk about this in the Naked Sex section.) Meaning, when we use our cues to tease each other a bit, we create a building of arousal from day to day. We begin to experience a sensuality that is romantic—that moves beyond the foot of the bed and begins to infuse our life with sensually loving experiences, consummated and not.

Your cues might be seeing your partner slowly undress, or watching him or her in a particular outfit, simple underwear, or lingerie. It might be a particular color that gets you going. Or seeing your husband standing in jeans with bare feet and a bare chest. It might be donning something elegant, or wearing something see-through. It could be a particular kind of kiss you offer, or just standing in the doorway and lovingly blocking your partner's path. It might be lying on top of each other—the physical connection of skin to skin. It could be dance music—swaying together in your living room for fifteen minutes—that gets you segued into your Naked Date.

But it's your job to find out what works—to experiment, to discover, and to try things out. To see what works, and to keep mental notes as a lover. This is an arena where it's perfectly okay to fail. You may try something that just doesn't float your lover's boat. But it's like that old adage about pizza: no matter how bad it is, it's never really bad. It's all good in the romantic neighborhood. Experimentation—touching and playing and attempting to arouse each other—all of it is good stuff when we love each other. So try and fail and try again, then laugh and enjoy and invent something else to try, until you kick in the door on something that sings and soars for your lover.

Take it on the road

Once you've got at least one romantic action or cue for each of you, you can broaden that experience and take it further than your living room and out beyond the foot of your bed. For instance, my husband likes to go shopping for shoes with me, and we get privately excited in public, just figuring out which high heels we might bring home to rock his world. I go shirt shopping with him, sit in the dressing room and watch him dress and undress. We're just applying and broadening our romantic sensual cues, taking them on the road with us, and having a little fun with them.

Sometimes we get dressed up in a suit and an evening dress, and then go to an elegant restaurant for a cocktail, just because it makes us—particularly me—feel special. When we do that we're using our clothing as a cue to be romantic.

It's a very sexy thing to be private in public—to present ourselves in lovely ways for each other's pleasure, in the company of others. It makes us see each other differently, and through the lens of others' viewpoints, which often, if we're truly being loving with our partner, makes us appreciate him or her even more. I always see my husband as handsome, but when we're out in public, and I see what a good person he is, too—how kind and open and strong and good he is with other human beings—I appreciate him more. I take celebratory ownership of him, thinking, "Wow. He's mine. Lucky me." And I find that experience sexy.

Early on in our first marriage, my husband hated parties and begged off whenever possible. He was painfully shy in those days, so we made a little pact: we would stick together at parties for the most part, and if I strayed into a conversation away from him for a while, he'd smile at me from across the room, inviting me to come back to him.

This became a sexual thing for us. At parties we'd hang out a bit, then I'd go chat with someone, and after a while he'd cue me from across the room with his eyes and a smile. It was like an invisible tug, the two of us being pulled together across a room as if by a string, and it was deeply private. It also turned us on.

Who knows why one thing rocks your sexual boat and another doesn't? Who can say why I'm wired to love having my partner look at me in outfits, and he loves to look? Who can say why, when we're arm in arm at a social event, we get hot for each other? I surely can't. We've just figured out that this is the way each of us ticks, and these are the things that make our sensuality wake up. We don't judge it. We just find it and use it and enjoy it.

That's the idea of the sensual cue.

Bite not the hand that loves you

That brings me to another salient point about romance. It needs to inform the way we talk to each other and the way we treat each other.

In my marriage, we have found that the more we engage in the Naked Date, and the more we add Naked Romance to our lives, the more we find a natural openness with each other. We call each other sweet names at home and in public. We're kind to each other. We have a terrific sense of humor about our faults, our shortcomings, and even our challenges as a married couple.

We didn't always have that. Our first time around, we were often withdrawn from each other, or distant or worried or agitated or edgy in our daily life with each other, and we didn't have a full-on kindness-and-appreciation ethic at all.

This doesn't mean we don't get pissed now, or irritable, or short with each other sometimes. Of course we do. It doesn't mean that we don't have disagreements or annoyances that have gotten under our skin for years. It doesn't mean that we're free of things we have to agree to disagree on—things that are largely unsolvable. Just like other couples, we have all of those things. That's the stuff of living with another human being—we are different animals, and we're never going to be exactly aligned.

What we try to do now is lead with an *active, romantic kindness.* To give the other person some breathing room. To listen. To not micromanage the other's feelings, or movements in the world, or belligerently insist on our own way. We try to notice that it's just us two; no matter what anyone else has to say about it, we either build a mutual road in the middle or we don't.

It doesn't take a rocket scientist to figure out that if one person is always driving the show—bullying, pressing, controlling, essentially not listening—then there's going to be trouble, and that's going to ding our romance, and certainly our sex life. If one partner is constantly trying to improve the other or can't stop making "suggestions" about how the other person should do things, that's going to zap the amorous feelings out of our romantic life, without doubt. So we have to lead with kindness if we want any romance at all.

One day we were at an art event talking to a couple we know. My husband started joking about backseat driving—something I am brazenly terrible about—and we were ribbing each other about it. I told a story about when we were on vacation and he drove the rental car over a huge rock where it wobbled and hung in midair, and I was so angry that I dug the gravel out around the rock until we shoved the car off into the dirt. (Not a smart move—I could have been hurt.) We both shook our heads and laughed at ourselves.

The jab was that he doesn't drive as well when he doesn't know the roads, so I *need* to backseat drive when he's at the wheel. His jab back was that the only reason I get to drive when we're traveling is because he lets me. It was a joking truth about a real challenge we have, and we were having a little light fun with it, gauging each other to make sure that while we were talking, it was landing on each other lightly, with laughter, as an honest but joking reveal of one of our foibles. It was gentle ribbing.

But the important part is our tone. We were laughing lightly at each other, and at our partnership. There was no edge. It's sexy to do that sometimes. To have a little fun with our faults and quirks, with the stuff that doesn't live in the sensitive danger zone. It makes us lighter with each other in public, and that makes us feel solid together, and then sexier, because we can weather stuff.

But that kind of teasing is also a delicate balance. So often it turns to edginess or meanness, with one partner seriously disparaging the other, and that won't work. Certainly, that scenario could have gone differently. If I knew my husband was sensitive or embarrassed about rolling the car over a rock, then it would not fuel my romantic life to bring it up, even in a joking way. The only reason it worked was because I knew he had a great sense of humor about the experience, and we had laughed about it together before.

My general rule is, if in doubt, say the *kind* thing, not the witty thing. I don't want to disparage my partner, I don't want to edgily poke fun at him in front of others, and I don't want to scald the feelings of fun and love and companionship we have built between us by being even a little bit mean.

We have to think about what comes out of our mouths and gauge the other person's capacity for teasing, and we have to experiment with what kind of tone—both at home and in public—works to keep our partner open to us. It's work, there's no doubt about it, to find the right balance. But that's what we're talking about here: finding the openings to love, to romance, and to marital fulfillment. So we've got to notice, and we've got to experiment, and we've got to try.

We don't want to bite the hand that reaches out to love us. We want to be generous, gentle, and thoughtful. That, all by itself, will go a long, long way to setting a daily stage for Naked Romance.

Propel your marriage into a Naked Romance

Romance is about more than just bodies. It's about seeing the other *person,* and being moved by another being—the person that we love. Surely, it's about continuing to love our partner—and many of us, no matter how long we've been together or what we've been through, will say that we do love our partner. But moving a marriage into a steady and long-term romance requires more than that.

We all know that we change and grow over the years of a marriage, both individually and as a couple, but it's our romance that helps us to stay deeply bonded to each other by sweetly and easily inviting us to focus on each other. It asks us to dig into the other's soul and body for what new inspiration we can find to love. That's the arc of a long-term love affair. That's the deepening—the "true love forever" stuff that we're all really after.

Romance lives, in a very primal way, in our physical selves, too. It lives in the sensuality of our skin, our breath, our sensations, and the awakenings of our sexuality. There's an artistry in the practice of opening to it, and we have to give ourselves a chance to keep the grace of it alive, to have the truest love experience we can have—to stay awake and to continue to find the inspiration for it.

As we said before, the inspiration for loving is not a spontaneous thing. Love and romance in marriage are slow to unfold and require open-ended, blocked-out hours that allow for allure, and sensation, and amorousness. That's the Naked Date/Naked Romance principle in a nutshell.

We all know that writers, painters, and sculptors can't make any headway if they only work when they feel "inspired." Waiting to feel a spontaneous urge to engage in creative work will never get them where they need to go. An artist works on having a *practice*—a regular bit of time set aside—with the understanding that creative inspiration shows up steadily only when regular, open-ended time is offered to the heart.

The same is true for romance. When those nonlinear, non-notification-oriented, non-checklist hours are offered us on a consistent basis, inspiration starts showing up right at its appointed hour. That's the point of offering ourselves naked romantic time.

We want those hours in marriage so that the slow and delicate movements of inspiration in love can appear, grow, and be built upon. We need to have a *practice* of setting aside time—even just an hour or two a week can do it—to get into our love life on a timely, regular, and dedicated basis. We want to propel our marriage toward a deepening—toward fun, and lightness, and joy, and arousal. Toward all of the things that make us delight in love.

We know the *David* statue wasn't carved in one sitting. The delight of the discovery came with work, effort, and time. It came with chipping away at the amorphous stone with hammer and pick, shaping the first bits of the revealed torso, trying and revising, adjusting and perfecting and polishing until the trust of repeatedly bringing hand to stone began to make that stone live.

These are the same joys of a long-term, loving marriage. Our willingness to try. Our set-aside time. Our sensual inspirations and our early efforts to apply them. Our time-in together, over weeks and months and years. Our failures, and the discoveries we make because of them. Getting up and trying again. The delight we take in carving out a bit of love that's satisfying and soul-warming. These are the gifts we want to give ourselves.

These are the gifts of a Naked Romance.

CHAPTER THREE
NAKED SEX

Set the stage for mutual intimacy

When I first began writing this book my husband sat me down, and with a little smile on his face asked, "Just how much of our sex life is going to be in this book anyway?" I laughed and said, "I really can't tell you. But since I'm talking about this from a personal perspective, some of it has to land on the page, right?" He looked dubious.

The next day he came home, put his hands on his hips, and said, "I thought about it, and I think you've got to talk about sex in detail. Our sex life changed dramatically from our first marriage to our second, so you've got to talk about what changed. This can't be one of those generalized, talk-around-it conversations or you'll never help anyone." I smiled and told him I agreed.

That said, this book is not designed to be a how-to sexual manual per se. (If you want terrific how-to guides, the best I've found are Lou Paget's books, *How to Be a Great Lover* and *How to Give Her Absolute Pleasure.*)

This book is about creating the environment for intimacy and pleasure, for setting the stage for mutual satisfaction, sensuality, and sexual fulfillment in marriage. It's about finding ways to get to the things we say are important, the things that truly enrich us and make us feel content, happy, and delighted. That absolutely includes our intimacy with our partner. So we're going to talk about how to get that satisfaction.

The other thing we're going to talk about is the development of *prowess* with our partner. Our object is to have an open, free-flowing, and accessible experience in sex with each other in our Naked Date so we will want to keep coming back to it. I call it having Naked Sex.

We said earlier that sex didn't always have to be part of the equation in a Naked Date. We can just get naked on a Thursday night at eight or a Saturday morning at ten and hold each other. But for lots of couples, being naked together will be a cue to get sexual, and we want that experience to be fulfilling for both partners (whenever sex happens), so that both are willing to have a Naked Date every week.

Naked Sex is about having the kind of intimacy that is mutual. It is not defined by the silly one-sided images of three-minute, slam-and-jam sex that we see in films and television. Sex for the long-term love affair is about the satisfaction of body and soul, senses and heart. That means, just like setting up a Naked Date and having some Naked Romance, we have to put a little effort into it. And we're going to talk about those efforts.

Make out

The thing we most often forget about our beginning efforts in sexual loving is that there was tons of ramp-up. We kissed for long periods of time before we went to second base. We held each other and pressed our bodies together passionately. We got a little close to the fire of touching in intimate places, and then we backed off or pushed each other away for a few seconds, and then dove back in. We were incrementally pushing toward something, and then pulling back, and the tension of that made us hot.

For many of us, when we were dating there was a prohibition against moving quickly into intercourse, so we had all kinds of sex play before we got there. Then, once we did *it*, as so many of the men and women I interviewed confirmed, it seemed like the drive to consummate just plowed over all of that foreplay to shoot straight for a finale. All of that delicious sex play was left by the wayside. And that's how many of us have been approaching our sex lives for years, particularly if we feel pressed for time. We head straight for a finale, without ever having a desire-building ramp-up. And it's a big mistake in a long-term marriage.

Once again, marriage is an animal that is slow to arousal. It has to separate itself from the crazy deadlines at work, the dead tree that just fell over in the driveway, the sick kids, and the refrigerator that just went kaput. It needs to take time out from the money worries, the concerns about aging parents, the arguments about who should clean out the garage. It needs, in essence, sexual warm-up time, and then set-aside exploratory time.

That means when we begin to approach our partner sexually, we have to do so with a spirit of drawing the other person out. We need to not expect that our partner will be instantly aroused, or brusquely move forward without sensitivity. In other words, we need to *stop taking overly direct routes in sex*, particularly if we want our partner to continue to desire us week in and week out.

When I was single, I had a boyfriend who was completely rough and fast in his sensual approach. He initiated roughly, he pressed quickly ahead, and there was no sensual ramp-up time at all. It was his way of trying to be fiery and passionate, and for a while I tried to meet him in that tone, but I became bored. It was intensely physical, but it was not fulfilling, and when he kept forcefully rushing even after I had asked him for something else, I not only stopped wanting to be sexual with him, I stopped wanting to be anywhere near him.

I was guilty of the same kind of rushing ahead in the early days of my first marriage to my husband, too. A lot of the time I didn't notice that he liked to draw out the anticipation of sex—to let desire hang in the air and build it—and I'd often press to get to the cliff-hanging heights before he had a chance to catch up. It wasn't sensitive on my part, and the driving nature of my need didn't allow for the lush, the exploratory, the tease, or the exquisite build of good foreplay. And that's all of the stuff we need in a long-term marriage.

Note that the need to build desire with touch is true for both men and women. The idea that men can just plow ahead without any need for foreplay does not hold true over the long term in marriage, and women can be just as guilty of prematurely pressing toward a finish line as the traditional male stereotype. So don't assume that gender excepts you from having to draw out your partner's arousal. It doesn't.

We have to find the right mix of *beginning* to draw passion out before we start with anything intense and pressing. Once more: when we're beginning to have sex, we need to *start at the beginning and take our time.*

Kissing is a hot and eroticizing way to begin. Making out, holding, pressing, dancing together, feeling each other's bodies, and lying on top of each other fully clothed before anything really gets going are all terrific steps in beginning an adult sexual encounter. And not just for two minutes, either. The more we draw these ramp-up moments out, the bigger the payoff we'll get when we get to the on-the-cliff peak of our arousal.

Let me put this in a clear and simple way: the lover who can take the time to kiss and to hold, to press and to pull back, and then press again, and who can revel in these moments and allow for a feeling of languishing in them can generally draw out his or her partner's sexual feelings. A lover who moves too fast cannot. Remember that the speed of mutual arousal in marriage is slow. That's just its nature.

The pace of your arousal efforts absolutely affects your partner's willingness to come back and be sexual with you the next time you want to be intimate, whether on your next Naked Date or any time. If the beginning of sex time feels like an assault on the senses instead of a provocation and an awakening, you will lose the willingness of your partner to frequent your body and your marriage's sex life.

Once you've mastered getting naked in bed with each other each week, try slowing down the pace. Take some time with kissing and holding, and maybe try not going straight for the bedroom. Hang out in the living room and kiss and roll around on the carpet on the floor. Press each other up against the wall. Dance or take just a few pieces of clothing off—not all of them. Stand in the shower with the curtain drawn back and let your partner watch you naked under the water. Take your time getting horizontal. Offer some time, some passion, some connecting, some variety, and some heightening experiences to your partner, long before any consummation takes place.

Know that these efforts don't have to be gargantuan or Casanova-like in length. Fifteen to twenty minutes of sex play before getting into direct stimulation can make all the difference in the world to our lover and can make him or her feel incredibly desired.

So kiss. Hold each other. Dance a little. Body-press a bit. Keep your clothes on for a while and touch *through* your clothes. Press your partner up against the living room wall and let your hands run up and down his or her body. Take your time. Let it all be part of a new erotic sex ethic.

In other words, *make out.*

A woman's body determines the pace

One of the most misguided things we've been taught by popular culture's images of heterosexual sex is that a man's needs determine the pace of sex; that the minute a man gets hard, intercourse is supposed to happen, and a woman is supposed to lay back and accommodate him. Abiding by this sexually regressive stance will totally ruin a marriage's sex life. That's an absolute.

First off, it's important for men to understand that a woman's physical arousal points are *not* as face-front as a man's: they are on the *inside*—not extending out of her body. Meaning that while a man and a woman are pressing and kissing, his arousal points are getting tons more stimulation than hers. She will not get aroused as fast as he does with straightforward body-to-body contact. That's just biology. He may already be hard and pressing against her, his breathing already quickening, while she's barely getting off the runway, with no particular touching offered to her erotic spots.

A good guide for men in relationships with women is this: *let the woman's excitement guide the pace of the sex.* Don't overpress. Don't rush toward intercourse, and don't let your own desire be the guide. If her breath is not reaching the same heights as yours, then you have work to do.

The point in sex is to draw out our lover. It's not for one person to *take* from the other; or for one partner to allow or *give in* to the other. That imagery is a dated Victorian sex ethic that has ruined more marriages over the years than is possible to count.

Even in its edgy, new-spin-on-the-Victorian, Netflix-special-series I'll-give-you-three-minutes-to-do-me-but-then-you've-got-to-get-out-of-here brazenness, sex that's one-sided is still just the same non-mutual, non-satisfying experience. We have to give that kind of thinking up in marriage if we want to have a happy sex life. Instead, we want to have a better understanding of what works in sex between partners and then apply it.

The biology of the thing

To get to the rhythm of the way we're wired as men and women when we're in physical love with each other, we need to understand our biology. Our sexual biology, that is.

(Note that in the next sections we'll largely be dealing with the biological dynamics of heterosexual marriages, though many of the mutual pleasure points will apply to same-sex marriages as well.)

As we just said, a woman's erotic zones are not face-front, while a man's zones are. So, if during the early amorous contact of male-and-female kissing and holding a man is getting much more stimulation than his female partner, what's he supposed to do? And what's she supposed to do to help move arousal along?

The answer is: *make contact.* For every press a man makes on a woman's body, for every touch she offers him on his visibly aroused flesh, he should be making sure she gets the same kind of contact—in equal or greater parts. That means using his hands or his legs or his belly or his mouth— or whatever inventions he can come up with to give her arousing and pressing contact. That means offering contact where it counts—right on her *mons,* the magic triangle of flesh that's filled with sensation—with both steady and light pressure, depending on what moves her most.

It also means that a husband needs to distinguish between the early amorous foreplay of touching and the later-in-the-act, more specific kinds of stimulation—that is, the kind of arousing touch that needs to begin with general pressing (think a flat hand versus too-fast and too-direct finger pressure on tender points) and a specific stimulating touch that's appropriate later for a take-me-over-the-edge release. These two kinds of touching are not the same thing, and a one-size-fits-all approach to sensual touch with no distinction or finesse will just make your partner retreat and back off.

Touch should feel like an awakening to begin with, then a mounting of feeling and sensation, and later on an intensification. That's how the body opens up fully.

For women, we need to understand that a man appreciates a teasing touch, a strong touch, and a stimulating touch, too, with mounting intensity, based on his rising excitement levels. We want to pay attention to those levels and adjust and offer what he needs. Just grabbing on and stroking him with no finesse and no understanding that he too has cycles of pleasure is not going to work.

Arousing touch and stimulating touch are different animals, and both partners need to be able to apply them appropriately and aptly.

Our biology has wired us into certain predictable arousal patterns— patterns that hold fairly true for many men and women. These are:

- A man's anatomy allows for more external contact, and often a quicker arousal, which can lead him to press for sex faster.

- A woman, with her erotic zones a bit hidden, tends to need attentive pressure on her erogenous areas to get sexed-up, and to catch up to where her husband is in excitement.

Our biology also determines the sex act itself. Women can (and this is obviously a generalization, not true for everyone) take longer to climax than men, and some men can often just release quickly without much steady work or attention from their partner. Based on that, many couples fall into the trap of letting the man drive the sex pace—letting him drive toward intercourse—which undermines the whole principle of mutual pleasure and deters the woman from wanting sex with her partner the next time. Doing that is going to rattle our Naked Date and make it fail, and we don't want that.

So let's take that challenge apart for a moment and think about our biology. Why are we wired like that? Wouldn't it be better if we were more equally arousable so that our levels of sexual drive would move toward each other at equal paces? Wouldn't that help us out a bit in marriage?

The answer is *no*.

A husband has what I call a "protector/provider" role with the wife he's chosen to be intimate with. I'm not talking about a husband's traditional role of providing for a family or a wife financially, which these days largely does not apply to the world of dual-working partners. I'm talking about a man's role in providing *pleasure* to his female partner in sex, based on the way we're biologically wired in heterosexual loving.

Meaning, if she takes longer to come, she needs to be able to trust him to be there for her. She needs to be able to *rely* on him—on his virile strength and control—while she builds in pleasure and hangs on the ledge a bit, and he needs to be able to provide that steadiness for her until she lets go. He needs to withhold his pleasure—and establish his virility and control—until hers is offered. That's how we build sexual trust between a husband and wife.

When a husband does this for his wife, her body relaxes with him. Her senses know that when he approaches her sexually the next time, there's satisfying pleasure in the works. She knows that her husband is masterful with her body, and that if she's willing to go to the vulnerable heights of hanging on a crazily aroused, oh-my-God-please-get-me-there cliff, that he will see her over the peak and into the sweet valley of release.

When I spoke with couples about the themes in this book, women often said that their sexual gratification comes from being pleased based on their own bodies' cycles and climaxes, but their husbands often reported that their pleasure comes *from pleasing her.* In other words, virility plays a big role in these men's sexual satisfaction, their own sexual self-esteem, and the couples' definition of what good sex is. That's important to know. That the satisfaction a husband provides in heterosexual sex is part of his *prowess,* and it feeds the marriage in a positive way.

When we weave that knowledge into how our biology works in our bodies, we can see that our sexual tendencies, when fully understood, actually serve us intimately in marriage. When a husband is expert in drawing out his wife's sexual desire—when he understands it and uses the slower pace of his lover's heat to masterfully draw her out—and he can *wait for her* long enough for her to take her pleasure, he will, as the husbands I spoke with confirmed, feel hot, aroused, and pleased by that. His prowess with her will allow him to freely let go into his own pleasure, too, but more importantly it will make her body trust him. It will allow her the freedom to build her desire and *know he will be there for her* until she's over the cliff and satisfied. He is providing for her, in the truest sense of the word.

The next time he approaches her, on their next Naked Date or another time, she is much more likely to open up to him because her body senses that his touch will bring satisfying pleasure. It's a very animal thing we're talking about here.

When a man doesn't do that, when he's constantly taking and pressing, and he's insensitive to her arousal cycles and doesn't provide satisfaction, she often stops wanting to have sex with him.

That won't work to have a satisfying sex life, nor will it work to support a regular Naked Date.

Bodies know things. If we've ever been insulted or hit or harmed by another, our body has an immediate reaction to that person's presence in the room with us. If we've been loved and adored and cherished by someone, our body has an immediate chemical reaction when we see them of ease, openness, and relaxation. The same is true in sex.

We want our bodies to be open to each other, and to stay open to each other, so that our Naked Date is a workable thing. So we have to let our biology serve us and bend to its will—not the other way around.

Moisture and more moisture

The other thing partners often overlook is the need for lubrication. Not the kind of lubrication that comes out of a jar—that's simple enough to apply when needed. I'm talking about the kind of lubrication that comes from foreplay.

In heterosexual marriages, I believe that a man's guide to moving forward should be his female partner's pace in arousal. Another way to say this is that his guide to moving ahead to more intense and direct sexual play should be *the drawing out of moisture.*

Dozens of the women I interviewed—as well as friends who have confessed this over the years—have told me that their partners will keep pressing for sex before they are anywhere near being lubricated. News flash, guys: that lovely apparatus you're sporting does not feel good inside without a little glide-and-slide to help it along.

What that means is that couples should have a guide with each other—a very practical understanding—about how long it really takes for the woman to get ready to have intercourse. That guide is moisture.

John Gray, the author of *Men Are from Mars, Women Are from Venus,* said on one of his books on tape that when he talked to men about how long they engaged in foreplay, they will, on average, say, "ten minutes." Privately, the man's female partner would tell him, "No. It's really about two minutes."

Ladies and gents, two minutes is *not enough* to generate heat—not enough to create the moisture that indicates a woman is aroused enough for intercourse.

Our biology is our friend here if we just pay attention to it. If we use the barometer of moisture to help guide both of us to the next heightened level, and we don't ignore the signs of the body that can help us tell if our partner is ready, we will have a much more fulfilling sexual experience—one that drives us back to our Naked Date each week instead of away from it.

That's how we continue to promote the willingness for a sexual encounter now, as well as a regular weekly sex experience later.

Be arousable

Yes, a man should be well aware of the nature of his female partner's arousal cycles, of what draws moisture from her intimate places, and what will work to make her *want him* inside her. We're not talking about when she's *willing* to have him enter her; instead, we want to align our sex with when her body says it's ready, when he's driven her excitement to a place where she *wants* and even *needs* penetration. A husband needs to know this, sense it, feel for it, and wait for it. That's prowess in its fullness.

What's a woman's responsibility in all of this? What's her role in helping arousal along so the act is pleasurable for both partners?

First, a woman needs to understand her own arousal and lubricating cycles. If that means practicing alone in her room until she knows what works on her body, then so be it. In sex, she needs to take responsibility for guiding her husband's hands to the places that will help her find excitement and gently aid him with pacing. She also, in my opinion, needs to not give in to being entered when she's clearly not aroused so her husband is not misled about how much attention she needs to be ready. But that means when it's not happening and he's pressing, she's got to not check out and help him along instead. That's the nature of intimacy: we have to be brave enough to share how we're really wired sexually.

As women, we want to both allow for arousal and seek it out. So, what does that mean in practical terms?

It means that we, as women, can't just sit back and expect our partner to draw out our desire from the dead zone. We have to bring something to the act. It's good for us and it's good for our marriage to have sex. It brings us close, it loosens us up, and it frees us with each other. So we have to be willing to be of service to the marriage by allowing for the pleasure of getting excited and by not holding back because we're blocking the vulnerability of being touched intimately. We want to let our body be available to our partner. That's the point of having Naked Sex in the first place: to open up, tell the truth, reveal ourself, and deepen our trust. To let pleasure take us someplace we didn't think we could go and to allow our partner to take us there.

Sometimes that's hard as a woman. We feel we've been shut up in our little ice cave of duty all week with nary a sexual thought in our head, and then we're supposed to just open up? And that's where our Naked Date can help us. Since we know when we're going to be intimate, we can prepare our bodies for love. We can ready ourself mentally, spiritually, and physically for our sensual time slot together. Meaning we have some real responsibility in guiding our thinking and our physicality to sexiness—in bringing something with us to the party.

For years I've sat in women's locker rooms and listened to women friends talk about dating men who they left for not having enough prowess with them sexually. A woman might say, "He wasn't anywhere near knowing what to do with my body." When I'd ask if she spoke up, asked for specific things she needed, or showed him specifically what to do, she would say, "I couldn't do that! I'd never be able to get the words out of my mouth! So I just stopped seeing him." This kind of thinking in marriage—where a wife is afraid to share or guide her husband in how to touch her—may not lead to one partner leaving the other, but it does usually lead to a shut-down of sexual experience between a couple. When a wife won't speak up, or won't be vulnerable enough to find a way to tell her husband what works, she shuts off the possibility for prowess to develop and usually closes off the future of any regularity of sexual experience with her husband. She avoids instead of telling him what works. We are not meant to grin and bear sexual touch that doesn't work for us.

And though I'm well aware that this land of speaking up to our husband (or wife) about prowess in sexual touch is filled with land mines, it is an absolute must if we're going to have the fulfillment we say we want. We can't keep pretending and then find the closeness we say we're after.

Certainly, we want our husband or wife to be able to arouse us—to have the basic skills of touching and pressing and drawing us out. If he or she is not doing that well, then we need to show our partner how.

We can't hide behind the fear of being vulnerably touched and still have a passionate, happy marriage. It's just not doable. We both have to do our part.

Same-sex fulfillment

In same-sex marriages the dynamic of mutual pleasure is not quite the same. The sexual gift in same-sex marriages is that both bodies are of the same gender, which can lead to an intimate understanding—one that often doesn't have to be explained—of how each partner's body works. But since human sensation is all over the map, and it's as varied as the number of bodies on the planet, that generalization is not necessarily always true.

One partner will usually, in his or her individuality, have some variety in how quickly or slowly he or she becomes aroused, or in the ways that arousal needs to happen. One partner may be more affected mentally by work stress or family issues or tiredness, and that will affect the couple's sexual excitement cycles. One partner may need more romantic connecting or ramp-up and foreplay.

But remember that marriage is marriage. It's slow to get hot and aroused, slow to separate itself from the daily workings of life. It needs a certain amount of time, relaxation, arousal, and stimulation to get it there. That's true for everybody in marriage, no matter the gender set-up.

In same-sex marriage, being there for our partner as his or her rising excitement occurs is just as important as with heterosexual couples. The ethic of learning each other's cycles, and not assuming that you already know them because you own the same equipment, is central to creating mutual satisfaction.

We can't just presume that because we're of the same gender that our bodies will work exactly alike or press the other partner to behave sexually the way we might find excitement. We have to listen and learn and reach out and meet our partner where he or she lives, no matter how the bodies are wired.

We want an ethic of being steadily there for our partner until we've lifted him or her into a pleasing and delightful arousal state, and then safely see our lover over the cliff into sexual release. We want a drawing out of love, of fulfillment and satisfaction.

What we're building is trust. Though our whacked, mind-bending popular culture sometimes has us wondering if the edginess of a new body is the way to find a startling release, it's actually trust, over time, with a partner who has mastery with us, that's going to bring that depth and thrill. Knowing we can be lifted into an amorous desire by our partner, and that he or she will see us all the way through—week in and week out—to the edge of our sexual heights, to the depths of what we're willing to explore—that's what will serve to heighten our love experience. It's what will build devotion, as well as the willingness to find new things together, and a genuine union of bodies and spirits.

Make your partner want to come back for more

How do we make our partner want to come back for more? How do we generate those feelings of willingness to be sexual each week in our partner's body so that our sex life—and our Naked Date—is preserved and well-supported?

First, we have to have an understanding of what works, over time, to draw our lover back. When we're pondering this question it's helpful to use a little analogy. Though I'm going to use the example of a heterosexual husband who is trying to understand the nature of why his wife often rebuffs him in sex, these ideas are also apt for women and same-sex partners. It's a simple analogy that can help us see the importance of satisfaction in loving.

Here it is. Let's say you love to eat and you're passionate about food. You love the smells, the tastes, the aromas, the flavors, and the textures of things melting in your mouth, and you adore the sweetness of taking the food all the way into your body. You love the arousal of eating, the tasting, and the swallowing sensations—the nourishment you feel when you're satisfied. Now, you're going to invite your favorite person—your wife—over for dinner. You lay out a beautiful meal: you both smell it, taste it, chew it, get aroused by it. But when it comes time to swallow and be satisfied, she's not allowed to swallow. Only *you* get to do that. You get the full satiated feeling in your stomach and your being, but she only gets the tease of it. She may say, "Oh, that's fine, I don't really need to be satiated," so you think you're on solid turf.

Then you invite her over for dinner again. You get to eat and be nourished and satisfied, and again she doesn't. Maybe she's occasionally allowed to fully eat the food, but most of the time she's not. After a while, she stops being interested in joining you for dinner, and you feel and sense her rejection. When you ask, "Why don't you want to have dinner with me anymore?" She may say something vague, like, "Oh, I'm just not a very hungry person most of the time." But the truth is, who would want to have dinner with you again? Who would want to get all juiced up and vulnerable to the sensual flavors of your meal and then not be allowed the satisfaction of it?

What's often going on when you have an ethic of nonmutual satisfaction in your sex life and your partner rejects you is this: *your partner's body senses danger with you and not pleasure.* In our example, her body is being asked to get half-aroused, half-way taken there, and it doesn't trust you to take her into her vulnerable, intense, tender, on-the-edge places, because it knows you'll often leave her high and dry.

Maybe she's also feeling pressured to get aroused at your rate of excitement instead of her own, and the insensitivity of that stance ends up turning her off. Her body *doesn't trust you*, based on her repeated experience with you. An instinctive danger-not-pleasure response will make her refuse you. It's simple self-preservation.

This dynamic is more traditionally thought of as a male-to-female experience, but it's apt for any couple in which one partner is regularly satiated in sex and the other is not. I've had husbands tell me that their wives refused to be touched after they've climaxed, claiming to be "too sensitive." The sex act just ended, with no attention to pleasing him.

Male or female, you cannot expect to have "sex for you" over and over again and have your partner continue to want you. You cannot rush the gates of physical contact, with no attention to the way your partner's arousal cycles work, take your pleasure without providing any, and expect a warm and willing response the next time you press your body up against your spouse.

You cannot be insensitive to the way she or he gets excited and not deliver regular sexual release, and then expect your partner to want to have a weekly Naked Date. You cannot be self-focused, telling her, "I only take three minutes to climax and you take twenty-five, so let's just do this quick," or, repeatedly telling him, "I need to stop; I'm too sensitive now," just when he's at his height and still expect that your partner's body will open to you the next time around.

Once again, bodies know things. A body knows whether your presence, close-in and close-up, is a satisfying thing or a dissatisfying thing. If there's danger in opening up to you—if your partner has to be prepared for the fact that it's a crap shoot whether or not her or his vulnerability with you will lead to any satisfaction—you're going to end up with a reluctant lover. Period.

My message to partners is this: don't engage in nonmutual sex in any regular way, particularly in your Naked Date. Just don't do it. You will ruin the desire cycles between you, and you will perpetuate the shutting down of one of you in your marriage. I don't care how long it takes for one partner or the other to climax. That's what the Naked Date is all about: setting aside time enough to have a mutually fulfilling sexual and sensual experience on a consistent basis.

We don't want to use the other person's body as a tool for our release. We want to be engaged with the other *person,* the way he or she is wired by God, by nature, and by the heavens, and then offer reverence, respect, and willingness in the sex act by giving pure and steady pleasure—the same pleasure we wish to have for ourself.

"Sex for Donny"

I have a friend who was dealing with a challenging situation in bed with her husband. She was frustrated and was having a hard time explaining why she was so agitated.

"It drives me crazy," she said. "It's always the same. There's sex for Donny, and then there's sex for me."

When I asked her what she meant, she said, "He gets excited, he's on me, and then when he's all through and he's lying there recovering, like an afterthought he thinks to roll over and do something for me. He'll sit up and say, 'Can I do something for you?' And I always feel like I should be grateful he's even thinking about pleasing me, but it's so mechanical. It feels like all the excitement and energy has gone out of it, and he's just there moving his hand on me, but his head is completely someplace else. We're not even close to having an experience *together.*"

I'm going to offer this thought as a guideline: if a husband is climaxing before his wife on a regular basis, there will likely be trouble. What I mean by that is simple: if a man is not providing pleasure for his wife with strength and prowess and expertise—with his ability to guide her into pleasure, allowing her to trust his steadiness until she's satisfied—she's going to stop wanting to have sex with him, and that's going to ruin any efforts to have a regular intimacy date.

The same is true for women. If a woman is not at all engaged in the way her partner's body works—if she's lying there, waiting to be entered without offering anything to eroticize him when it's his turn to climax—then he's going to be less excited about the prospect of sex with her the next time.

If a couple is particularly skilled in bed and has lots of sexual experimentation at their disposal, it's great once in a while for a wife to say to her husband, "This is all for you, babe," and then let him pleasure her later another way, after he's climaxed. But on a steady basis, particularly in your Naked Date, if you're a man and you want your female partner to want to come back for more, I lovingly suggest that you please her *first*. If you're a woman, you need to keep your head and your desire in the act when it's time to please your husband.

We all know that there's nothing worse than feeling that your partner's energy to please you has drifted off into the ethers, and he or she is just going through the motions because they're supposed to. The object is to *stay in*.

The simplest thing I can offer on this count is to *breathe with your partner, breath for breath*. When you stay connected to each other's breathing patterns, it will guide you both to levels of excitement that work together. It will help you both stay connected to the oneness that good sex brings. Then, once you find the gift of assured mutual pleasure, of the expertise of a providing partner, and once your bodies both trust that mutual satisfaction *together* is what will happen in your Naked Date every time, you can throw out the rule book and go for broke.

JoBeth and Cameron

When I first met Cameron and JoBeth, they claimed everything was going well for them. Since their kids were grown and gone, they had experienced "a new acceptance" with each other, according to JoBeth.

When we began to talk about the specifics of intimacy and how it had played out in their lives over a thirty-year marriage, JoBeth clammed up. "I don't want to talk about that," she said snippily.

Cameron flushed red for a moment. "She doesn't want you to know that she won't have sex with me anymore," he blurted out.

JoBeth was clearly angry with his revelation, but she didn't leave as we started to talk about it.

"Look, all of my women friends over fifty say the same thing. We did all that. We're done with it, and we shouldn't have to anymore," she said.

Cameron nodded his head in her direction. "That's where we are."

After a few simple questions about whether that stance was a happy and contented choice for them both, Cameron spoke up: "No it's not. Truth be told, I love her, and I still want her."

When I pressed a little more, JoBeth said, "I just don't have the desire."

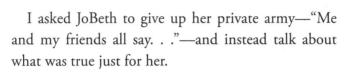

I asked JoBeth to give up her private army—"Me and my friends all say. . ."—and instead talk about what was true just for her.

The lack of desire is a common challenge for couples, but I wanted to know if there had been a "what happened"—a term I use in my coaching that relates to an event that shut something down. Cameron explained that when their first child was going off to college, JoBeth had an emotional affair with her guitar instructor. No intercourse took place, but some sexual affection (lingering hugs and holding) did, as well as daily talking and confiding, and some kissing.

"I feel like ever since then she's been punishing me for making her stop," Cam said. "We really stopped having a sex life then, ten years ago."

They had been to therapy, aired their feelings, dealt with their hurt, and decided to stay together, but they had not been able to get back to creating desire between them.

I asked JoBeth what the other man had given her that had ramped up her desire. "It wasn't the breaking the rules part," she replied. "He really *listened* to me. Just listened. We talked about all kinds of things every day. And I got close that way and wanted to be close."

That was a huge *bingo* for us in what we could create, practically, to help them.

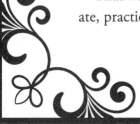

Cameron seemed to be easy to talk to and was not the least bit short with JoBeth. I asked if she felt Cameron had the capacity to listen to her. "He's just not interested, that's all," she said.

I explained to Cameron that JoBeth's relationship to sex, or any kind of intimate touching or emotional closeness, was predicated by *being known.* Sharing intimately was a key for her in allowing the gates to drop down so she could be emotionally and, I was guessing, physically vulnerable.

Meaning that if he wanted to have a sexual relationship with his wife, he had to learn a new kind of foreplay—talking and sharing—something that, as an engineer, might not come naturally to him.

"I think I'm a good listener, most of the time," Cameron said. In response, JoBeth rolled her eyes: "Please. You've had your head in a book or a newspaper for thirty years."

I asked them to stop bringing up *anything* from the past, including past ways of behaving, and to be willing to *start from today* to implement some new suggestions.

I suggested they try sitting down at a set time once a week to have a Couch Talk—thirty uninterrupted minutes to talk and listen to each other. This would give JoBeth a chance to share what's really going on with her and to hear what's going on with Cameron.

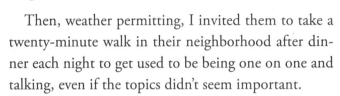

Then, weather permitting, I invited them to take a twenty-minute walk in their neighborhood after dinner each night to get used to be being one on one and talking, even if the topics didn't seem important.

Two weeks later, they checked in. "I can feel we're getting somewhere," JoBeth said. "We're even holding hands when we walk. Silly, but it makes me feel really good."

I asked them both to start querying each other in their talks to show interest—to not fake it, but to come up with genuine questions or ask for details on each other's stories, feelings, or comments. The upshot to the guidance was *no fixing, just listen, query, and comment kindly.*

After a couple of months, they were ready and willing to try the Naked Date. JoBeth knew it was going to be tough for her to be sexually vulnerable again, and Cameron agreed it would be intense for him, too. I asked them to prepare for intimacy with themselves solo and to do it differently—to arouse themselves in some way other than they had before in their solo sex—and to *not climax.* In other words, to try some sensual, slow pleasure for the sake of it.

I asked JoBeth to keep a journal of sexual thoughts, so she'd have access to them when she was being intimate with Cameron, and to get herself some lubrication that she liked. If they had full-on sex the first time, fine, but it didn't need to happen.

We talked quite a bit about the mutual pleasure principles in this chapter, about Cameron waiting for JoBeth's pleasure, and about finding varying routes to arousal on each other's bodies.

After a month, they had successfully gotten back in bed together, with both experiencing a good, long sexual ramp-up and fulfilling release.

JoBeth said, "I'm surprised at how much having sex together has taken the edge off. I've stopped being angry at him for stupid things, and I feel close for the first time in years. But what's most surprising is that now that he's really listening to me, I find I want sex with him. It makes me cry that I missed that for so long."

"I would have done just about anything to have my wife back, but I didn't know what to do," Cameron stated. "It's a gift to get this back now, when I thought we'd never have it again. I'm grateful."

"I'm okay, honey"

There's a stereotype in our culture that women are less sexually charged than men. But what I believe is this: men have been given more permission to be sexual than women have. Girls, when growing up, were historically assigned to be the gatekeepers of warding off sex, and boys were given the latitude and social acceptance of having sexual thoughts and experiences. Women were not allowed to admit to the sexual feelings, thoughts, and experiences they actually had, and that repression is still with us.

In my opinion, that's why so many teenage girls today who are in the process of their own sexual awakening have identity issues. Good girl/bad girl stereotyping still brands a girl who is sexual as "bad," and a girl who is not as "good." Young women who are exploring their sexuality still have no good imagery to attach themselves to if they want to have a normal progression of sexual awareness and growth in their early sexual awakenings—and they are unlikely to get this guidance from the adults in their sphere.

Though that's changing, it's a problem if we're still, as adult women, holding onto those girlhood gatekeeper mores of warding off sex (or not admitting that we're as sexual as we are) in our marriage.

Boys, by turn, were expected to know what to do, as if by some intuitive psychic power, with no training and no effective information offered. That means lots of men entered their marriages with no clue about how a woman's body works, and then carried the self-focused sexuality of their early years into their long-term marriages. In other words, driving straight to intercourse, with no idea how to make the whole experience pleasurable for both partners.

We wouldn't think to withdraw mathematics from a young person's entire schooling years, and then expect them to jump into it when they reach a marriageable age. But that's what we do with intimacy. As a society, we offer few skills, scant teachings, and very little encourage-ment to help our kids experience their awakening sexuality as normal, or to prepare them for acquiring the skills they need to be a good sexual partner in marriage. That means many women and men have issues finding their way sexually and sensually once they're married adults.

But those overly ingrained mores don't mean that women, particularly the way we're wired biologically, are actually less sexual in body and spirit than men. In fact, in marriage, many women (and so very many who I interviewed) have the same challenges with their male partners going asexual on them that men sometimes complain about with women. That is, domesticity can tend to deaden their male partner's desire. (This can be just as true for same-sex marriages.)

That's exactly why we need a Naked Date. We need a special time set aside to open up, to be sexual and sensual for the pleasure and delight of both of us. When we do that, we allow for the ignorance of all of that historical "women are not that sexual" or "men should always drive toward sex" nonsense to fall away so we can breathe in the pleasure we're entitled to.

Sometimes, when heterosexual sex has been unequal in mutual pleasure for a long time, a woman will block her partner's willingness to help her find satisfaction by saying, "That's okay, honey. Don't worry about me. I'm fine."

I urge you not to fall for that kind of avoidance in your Naked Date. When one partner is physically satisfied in sex regularly and the other is not, the unsatisfied partner will—almost without fail—start to avoid intimacy. Her or his body will not feel safe enough to keep engaging in half-arousal, half-excitement, halfway-there titillation with no safe and sure guiding to a release. That's just the way our intimate bodily trust cycles work.

As women, though, we have a responsibility to not hide behind the untruths like, "I'm just not that sexual," or "That's okay honey, I'm just fine without you pleasing me." We absolutely cannot fake pleasure or climaxes—that's just hanging any efforts we're making to have a loving, honest, open sexuality with our partner. Faking it is an intimacy issue, just like pretending that your pleasure isn't that important; it's checking out rather than telling the truth about how we're wired or what we need.

When we engage in falsity in sex, we go down a dark, emotional road, privately engaging in thoughts that our partner is inept or that we'd rather have someone else in our sex life. Those are dangerous thoughts. Instead, we want to be courageous enough to give up those false stances and make a brave and willing effort to show our partner what works for us. We have to give up all of that childish sexual nonsense we were taught about warding off advances and not being able to admit we're sexual and take our pleasure into our own hands—literally and metaphorically—and then empower our spouse's hands.

Everyone can stand a little pleasure once a week, and we know without doubt that it's good for our marriage. The truth is, we're all human here. Bodies are not that complex. There are only so many positions and poses and rhythms and uses of the equipment we have, and we are *all* fully capable of learning how to use it well. It's not rocket science. With just a little information and a little practice, sex can become a heightened and mutually satisfying river of pleasure that we delight in dipping into each and every week.

I know this sounds like I'm proposing a heavy focus on climaxing in sex. As we move deeper into this chapter, we'll broaden that thought to allow for more flexibility and experimentation, fewer guideposts and more free association. But to set the stage for a successful Naked Date—to build a rock-solid foundation of week-in and week-out intimacy—the kind that brings closeness and passion to our marriage—we have to have a *mutually* fulfilling sensual experience.

That's what makes us want to come back to our partner again and again for our Naked Date, and that's why we're setting the parameters for that here.

Why refusals hurt

Refusals—when we approach our partner for intimacy and we get put off—hurt. They won't wound us to the core when offered once in a while, but if they happen all they time, they'll send us in the other direction, away from our partner.

When we begin having a Naked Date, we create a baseline for intimate communion, closeness, and sex. That baseline often helps us to heal the issues with refusals, which can occur when one partner approaches sexually and the other rebuffs, claiming to not be in the mood.

The Naked Date creates a time to *get* in the mood, to be available to being sexual and intimate, and that helps each partner relax, knowing there'll be time and there will be willingness to get naked and erotic with each other. That helps the sexually anxious person relax, and it also helps the sexually reluctant partner wake up to sensuality by providing some ramp-up time. It's a commitment to be available to each other, and that assists our loving.

When one partner is seeking sex much more often than the other, the pressure of that need can rattle a marriage. Do you remember the hilarious scene from the classic film *Annie Hall* when Woody Allen's character, sitting in his analyst's office, is asked, "How often do you two have sex?" "Hardly ever!" he replies. "Three times a week." Diane Keaton's character, in her own analyst's office, replies, "Constantly! Three times a week." Though the scene is humorous, it speaks to a lack of agreement between the couple that's eating away at what was once a fine connection.

The Naked Date serves to ameliorate all of that angst about when, how often, and how much. We set a time, we agree to show up, and then we get close. But over and above our commitment to get naked once a week, we want to find a balance between being available to our partner *sometimes* for random and unplanned intimacy, and allowing for solo pleasure, which we can agree is our partner's prerogative if his or her need for release requires attention more often than ours. Yes, we're trying to create an environment of love, affection, sensuality, and mutual eroticism so that we're accessible to it, but our needs will not be the same all the time. So we need to have a plan for that with an agreement that allows for our differences, yet still keeps us close.

First, to find that agreement we want to balance requests for intimacy well and kindly. If one partner asks and the other continually refuses, the asking partner will often get hurt enough to distance himself or herself rather than talk about their feelings. That's the way we are as humans. That's why it's a good idea to have clear agreement. Something like, "Hon, I love our Naked Date, and I'll enjoy a bit of spontaneous eroticism once in a while, too—probably on weekends when I'm not stressed—but if you need more than that, I support you in taking care of yourself solo."

Being available, and not wanting to hurt our partner's feelings, doesn't mean we have to say yes every time we're asked either, particularly if a partner is offering us no other affectionate contact besides a sexual advance or if we sense he or she is using sex to make up for other feelings of inadequacy; e.g., clinging to sex for self-esteem rather than dealing with an inability to get a job or face some other life challenge. This is more common than we might expect.

Our goal is to find balance and agreement by noting what our desire cycles are like, and then allow for those cycles to be addressed.

In my own marriage, some weeks our world is so clamorous that we're lucky just to get to our Naked Date. Other weeks our Naked Date sparks a whole weekend of spontaneous openness and sex, eroticism and play. Sometimes I'm the one with more desire beyond our weekly sensual time and I need to take care of myself while my husband is distracted or busy, sick or worried. Sometimes, it's him. But no matter what hellfire or sweetness the week rains down on our heads, we always honor our Naked Date together, and try each weekday to engage in little acts of kindness, affection, closeness, and little bits of sex play to prime the pump.

We give up curt refusals by having agreement and understanding, a willingness to play with and romanticize each other, and a solid weekly Naked Date that satiates our souls, bodies, hearts, and minds.

When the body shuts down

When my husband and I were separated and unraveling into divorce, we got together for several weekends and had sex, attempting to magically put the glue back into our flailing marriage. It didn't work.

Our sex became sex-for-me. He'd get aroused and please me, but when it was time for him to let go, he wouldn't climax. His inability to let me please him drove me crazy. His body would only go so far with me, and since we were about to be divorced, that made sense. But in my warped sensibility at the time, I thought I could solve issues by using sex as glue. He felt this, and his body refused to let go to me. There was nothing either one of us could do about it. There was not enough trust between us to find real release, and his physical and spiritual senses knew it.

If I had had a bit more wisdom, I would have figured that out. I was not safe to him then. We weren't addressing what was wrong, and my press to go over the edge with him sexually had some falseness to it. Both of us, by engaging in the act, were asking each other's hearts to pretend we weren't hurt and scalded. We were asking each other's bodies to open up when our bodies knew better; we couldn't be fully aligned when there were piles of issues between us that were breaking our hearts.

When one or both partners shut down, and when there's serious trouble over marital breakdowns, the best thing we can do is stop pushing for sex. If the sex is affected, that means there is a large and smelly elephant in the room that needs addressing—usually having to do with some other issues way beyond intimacy. That elephant needs to be deflated and shooed out the door, and then some fresh air needs to be let in before intimacy can flow once again. Remember, intimacy is a reflection of how we're doing in our relationship, not vice versa.

Angling for sex when there are huge things amiss can feel like sticking a knife into a painful wound. And, yeah, sometimes we push for it anyway for the edgy thrill it gives us. Sex can be a great turn-on when there's trouble because there's desperation in it—meaning, we don't know if we'll be together ever again, and that uncertainty can fuel some heat. But later it brings painful emotions, which the body stores up, so the next time there's an opportunity for sex, it may very well shut down on us.

The message here is: don't pretend that sex can make up for what's needed in the arena of communication and working through serious problems. Good sex flows from smooth and contented communication, from agreement and willingness, from effort and working through things, and from trust.

Mix it up

Beyond the mutual satisfaction issue, there's another element that helps to keep our partner coming back for more: *variety*.

Usually in marriage we have our go-to stuff with our partner: the things that we know will arouse, stimulate, and satisfy our lover. And we're going to rely on those things a lot over the course of years. We've learned a little something about how he or she works. We know that if being on the bottom isn't increasing her excitement level, we can flip her on top and that will do the trick. We know that brushing his chest lightly with our fingernails, and then a little more intensely, will quickly take our slow and steady rocking up a notch for him.

But to make things continue to spark, to keep things interesting, we have to mix up the way we get there and the way we use the strategies we have. In other words, we need to vary the rhythms, the directions, the lines, the pace, the order of things, and the way we get to a grand slam.

That's what so beautiful about the Naked Date. It's discovery time. It's time carved out from the week that gives us an opportunity to be inventive and explore.

It's a lot like the time we might set aside to be creative. In my book, *How to Be an Artist,* I note that engaging in artistry requires undisturbed hours to explore—particularly when we're first working with an idea and need to improvise a bit; we need to try things, and then pull it apart and reconstruct it, until we know we've got something that really works. And we can't give our soul creative permission to explore unless we offer ourself some regular, steady hours so our inspiration has a chance to surface and be built upon.

The same is true for loving.

If we're not planning time for exploration, we can drift into boredom. If we know the exact same things are going to happen whenever we close our bedroom door, we can get frustrated with the sameness of the thing and stop wanting it altogether. And we don't want that—not for our own spirit and body, and not for our partner's.

The Naked Date is magical because it gives us the ability to *plan* for things. Sexual things. To think about them, and then connect the dots of exploration in our brain and body. To ready ourself to engage in them. It gives us time for inspiration to find us, and then frees us to *play* and explore.

Once we're in the act, we don't have to rush. We can languish over our partner and revel in the event. Paced fast or slow, tender or intense, we've got time to experience all of it.

There's another thing that our intimacy date offers: when we have some time parameters to be together, and we honor that time week in and week out, we tend to get a little looser. That may mean having a little romp on the bed, then getting up in the middle of the act and dancing naked in the hallway. It might mean having sex standing up in the kitchen, and then landing on the living room floor. It might mean wandering from room to room, christening each.

The upshot is, when we have dedicated time, we tend to feel freer. As we get used to the Naked Sex principles, and we start to trust that our Naked Date time will be there for us consistently, our creative sexual inspiration tends to show up at the appointed hour, too . . . then the fun really begins.

There's all kinds of things we can play with sexually that won't require us to be overly inventive or herculean in our efforts. Maybe it will be for-your-eyes-only clothing or experimenting with photography (and then printing that little keepsake photo to keep in our wallet). We might want to seek out our partner's favorite music and then dance to it with each other—or for each other. We may want to play in the bath or the shower or get out in nature someplace private enough to have a little romp in the woods. These suggestions don't take much to implement and can be done close to home. If we're inventive, we may want to find something edgier or more extravagant. It's not particularly important to be elaborate, but we want to vary what we do to invite newness and bodily delight.

Then, we also want to mix up the way we get from *A to B*. Meaning, we want to vary the routes we take in our touching.

For example, to be a good vinyasa yoga teacher, I have to work with the limited number of existing yoga poses, and then mix up the rhythm and the order of those physical shapes, building on them to create a challenging *flow* from pose to pose that slightly surprises the student. Yes, I have some set series of poses that I work into my classes, allowing students to anticipate some things, but I don't want them to be able to anticipate everything. To try to find balance in a series of poses we're not used to is part of the fun and part of the challenge.

The same is true for lovers. We have to work with the limited number of poses possible in the sex act, and then play with the ways the body gets aroused to surprise and delight our partner. And even when the touch and the pose may be familiar, the way we get there needs to vary and can benefit from our invention and our creativity.

The easiest way to find this variety is to simply change the order of what you do. Break it up. Stop in the middle and do something different. Try one position for three minutes, then try another. Stop in the middle of early intercourse, pull back, and do something oral. Pause and do something with your hands. Tease a little with penetration then get up and move to another room.

Once we've set aside Naked Date time, we want to *just play*. To relax, enjoy, discover, invent, take our time, and satisfy. That's the joy of mixing it up.

Have Some Sex that's not consummated

One of the great gifts of playfulness is to be able to engage in sex acts that are not consummated. Does that sound like a contradiction to what we've been talking about regarding mutual pleasure? It's not.

Our Naked Date time is for mutual fulfillment, but once we get that train rolling on a regular basis, it's fun to have some sex play at other times that doesn't necessarily have to lead to full-blown sex or climaxing.

We're talking about the ability to arouse each other a little bit and not drive directly to a finish line. To tease a little, and then walk away. To walk out into the world now and then hyped up on each other's skin and breath, tingling with arousal, having done nothing about finishing it off. This kind of play is about being electrified, literally, for a few sweet moments before we move into our daily responsibilities. That means—you guessed it—getting a little juiced up just for the sake of getting juiced up.

When we enter this phase of sexual exploration together we're moving into what I call "The Adult Disneyland." It's a land of sensuality that doesn't stop at the foot of the bed, that's not bound by the hours of our Naked Date. It's a way to create a continual sense of sweetness and joy in our contact together—kissing and holding and touching, maybe just for moments, getting oral or rocking each other a bit for one or two minutes just for fun, and then parting— high on each other. It's a land of evocative touch and pleasure, of being connected to what's mature and adult in a long-term, hot, passionate, love affair.

Sexual awakenings bring more sexual awakenings. That's how we're wired as human beings. Yes, there's satisfaction in release, and usually when a fulfilling release occurs with our partner we're not immediately pressing to jump right back on top of him or her with the same need we had before a climax. Our bodies have a relationship to being filled sensually after a satisfying sex act, just like when we feed ourselves. But when we're intimate on a regular basis, and that intimacy is satiating, our bodies stay open to more sensation. And we can take advantage of that in marriage to offer each other a little bit of here-or-there sex play or closeness just for fun.

We want to arouse each other just for the hell of it, simply for the delight of being turned on. This isn't sex for one person, or for the person who can come faster than the other. This is *unconsummated* sex play, or not-all-the-way-there play, which means no one is climaxing. It's purposeful play to arouse and ignite the senses, to make our partner move through his or her day with an erotic sense of our skin deep inside their own. It's a little tease to keep us aware and alive, to keep the sex juices flowing.

It might be as simple as a pressing, arousing touch over the bathroom sink in the morning or just walking around naked together at home and caressing each other as we pass in the hallway. It might be a bit of oral play or pressing our bodies up against the bedroom door while fully dressed. It might be a bit of direct sex play, and then a pulling back before anyone's excitement starts to rise. I like to think of it as erotic touch in one- to three-minute intervals.

There's another aspect of this kind of sex play that's terrific: it builds more trust. If satisfying our partner regularly is the ultimate in confidence and belief in our sensual communion, then unconsummated sex play is an act of that faith. It requires trust to arouse each other *just to be aroused.* To revel in that act of sensual hanging-on-a-cliff, and then take those awakenings into our day, alive with the spirit of our partner in our body and our soul, is a grand and glorious thing. It deepens our sweetness with each other, our access to each other's bodies, and our trust with each other.

Bringing each other the smells, the tastes, the skin-to-skin sensations of a simple, brief act of unconsummated intimacy can lift up our day in a way that is so sweet that we find ourself smiling all day long, rich with the tenderness, heat, and arousal of our partner's ardor.

And that, my friends, is a good day.

Show and tell

So, let's say you've been a bit of wallflower in asking for what you want in bed, or you've gotten into a routine that's lost its sheen. Or maybe your partner is moving too fast for you or not touching you in ways that help you get into the act. And let's say that's getting in the way of you wanting to commit to a weekly Naked Date. What can you do?

You have to unequivocally *tell* him or her, whether by body language or in words; you have to either show or tell. That's the point of intimacy—to be naked in body and soul. To let your lover in on how you're wired so he or she can please you.

Trust me when I say that we each know how delicate this realm is—both for our own heart and our partner's sense of prowess with us—and we all tremble at the thought of telling our lover that we want something new or we want something *else*.

What we really want is for our partner to just *know*, to sense into our being and just intuit what we want, as if by magic. We don't want to have to physically place his or her hands in the right spot, with the right pressure, or try to correct the rhythm, or *talk* about it. (Good God, no!)

Truly, that's just not fair. If we're not willing to express what we want, then how can we expect our partner to figure it out? We have to woman-up and man-up a bit here, and be a little braver for the sake of our marriage.

When at all possible, we want to begin by using *actions, not words*. This is the best thing to do when we're in the sex act itself. Nobody wants to be in the middle of intimacy and have our partner say out loud, "You're not doing it right. Will you *please* just move your hand to the left?!" That's not going to get us the attentiveness we're longing for, and it's just not nice.

That brings up another thought that will help us across the board in communication. That is, we have to speak up or guide our partner to a different way of touching us before we get irritated. We're all extremely delicate in the sexual realm where our confidence is concerned, so we can't wait until whatever is happening is so agitating that we snap at our partner.

Let's say our partner is pressing or rubbing but is way off base. Keeping in mind that we're working to match our lover's excitement breath for breath, we want to stay in the intimate energy of the act and gently guide our partner's hands or hold onto hips to adjust the speed, or move fingers from an intensely stimulating touch to a more serene pressing touch, or vice versa.

This is an important note for women in particular. Take charge for a moment, but do it with kindness, and do it with pleasure. Don't be passive. Passivity is another way of checking out. We don't want that.

To stay inside the drive for excitement while at the same time giving ourself the dignity of a pleasurable experience by *participating* in it is the theme. Remember that in heterosexual sex men report feeling satisfaction when their partners are pleased, and women report feeling pleased when they are satisfied in their own bodies. We need to benefit from that dynamic and grab the wheel to help guide our partner to our own excitement; to help drive the car of our own pleasure for the sake of the relationship.

Key into it. Guide your self and your partner to it. Open your breath and your body and your secret ways of getting excited. That's the idea.

Think of it this way, we want to do everything in our power to assist in making our sex act a *coupling of two*. A mutually satisfying discovery of two. That's what sex is supposed to be.

Words, words, words

If we're guiding while in the sex act with our body language, our hands, and our breath, then it's a good idea to be verbal only in monosyllabic words. Words like, "yes," "good," "there," and "more," work much better than: "That seems like it's really working for you. Is it?" Sex is not a diatribe, and it's not an intellectual enterprise. Even when you're trying to guide your lover to be more adept and expert with you, it's a good idea to stay inside the act by using sex words.

This seems really obvious to some of us, but to others it's not. I once dated a man who was constantly commenting, in full sentences, on what we were doing together during the ramp-up to intimacy, and all it served to do was distance me. It was like he was observing the act instead of participating in it. (He was a psychologist, funnily enough.) It bothered me so much that we stopped dating.

So don't mistake sex for a conversation; it's not—unless you're both very into bold and provocative sex talk, but that's a whole different animal.

Sex is an experience of sensations that relies on the intuition, the senses, and the intelligence of the body. So whatever you're doing to guide or direct or respond needs to stay in the realm of breath and passion.

Sometimes, no matter how hard we try to guide with our hands and our body language, our partner just misses the message. That doesn't mean he or she doesn't love us or isn't capable of learning. It means—straight-up—that we have to say something. We have to speak up.

How do we get the stuttering, imperfect words *out* of our mouth to tell our lover to try something else? We need to ask, but we need to ask wisely.

What does that mean? It means we don't stop in the middle of sex and have a conversation about it (unless everything has broken down). And we don't say, "Hey, I need to talk to you," as soon as the act is over, and then launch into what just went wrong. We don't want to have something negative to say each time we engage in intimacy, as if we're grading our partner and handing out a "D" or an "F."

Here's the best way I know to tell our partner we need something new or different in sex. Wait at least a day or two after sex before you have the discussion. Then, apply what I like to call "The Love Sandwich." First, you say something nice, then you speak your business, then you finish with something loving. Simple, direct, to the point, with not too much rambling or getting lost in the weeds, if at all possible. Try to stick to just a few sentences. I like to write mine down so I don't end up rambling or skirting the point.

Here's an example: "Honey, I love it that you want me every week, and that your desire for me is so steady and true. I really adore that. I'd like to ask you for something in sex. When we're first kissing and getting warmed up, can you spend another five or ten minutes touching me between the legs, pressing with a flat hand, so I can get as hot as you're getting? I would love that. You're so sweet to me, and I so enjoy getting excited with you."

The way this works is simple:

- You're approaching your partner during a non-sexual time and expressing something intimate in a non-charged way.
- Since you're not in bed, your partner's feelings are not tenderly near the surface the way they often can be in sex, so you're likely to be heard more clearly.
- You can discuss details in specifics without any pressure to perform what you're asking for, which gives your partner a chance to think about how to implement what you're asking for.

If a demonstration is required, then go into the bedroom and show your partner what you're talking about, but my loving suggestion is to *not* have sex then. Stop what you're demonstrating, even if it's getting you aroused, and wait until the next full-on sexual experience. Otherwise the two of you run the risk of testing and grading each other—giving a "B," or a "C," or an "F"—and that's not going to aid you on your next Naked Date or sex encounter.

Let sex be sex, and talk be talk, and let demonstrating what you want be a simple show-and-tell, and then back off and let your partner figure out how to integrate the new information you've offered into his or her sexual toolbox for another day. That's my suggestion.

The upshot is, when we're talking or demonstrating, we want to preserve our partner's ability to implement what we're asking for on his or her own terms. Yes, we want to speak up for our own pleasure, but then let our lover find his or her own way to us without micromanaging.

When our partner starts to put our requests into practice, we want to be careful not to dissolve into Am-I-doing-it-right conversations during sex. Fall back on nonverbal guiding, body language, and monosyllabic words or sounds (e.g., "mmm" and "yes") versus full-on sentences like, "Well, that's sort of it."

The way we use words is incredibly important to our sex, and especially our Naked Date, for the simple reason that we're trying to build regular, satisfying intimacy into our marriage every week. These suggestions are the best ways I know to preserve our partner's dignity and open ourselves up to the truth of our own pleasure with him or her.

Think sexy thoughts

When we think about personal responsibility in marriage, we rarely talk about what I call "thought responsibility." In marriage, we usually wait for our spouse to do something to us to draw us out—romantically, sensually, sexually—and we expect that those actions will then turn our thoughts to sexiness.

But what if we have a responsibility to think sexy thoughts? To bring something to our marriage that we can draw on from inside our very nature that keeps us open to the land of sensation and loveliness and the eroticism of life? I believe we each have that responsibility.

Thought responsibility means attending to sensual images and ideas in our hearts and minds and holding them there, like a lovely cache of secrets, that we can draw on to ramp up to lovemaking. Taking our thoughts to the eroticism of the sensual things we've witnessed and experienced during the week can help us get in the mood.

We're not talking intrigue behavior, hitting on other people besides our spouse or pretending we're with another person in bed, trying to get a hit off someone else to sexually charge up our body. We're also not talking about cruising for sex images all week long that are outside the realm of our marriage. Those behaviors are intimacy issues and won't help our sex life or our devotion.

What I'm talking about is noticing what passes us during the week that awakens our sensuality, how it sparks our fantasies, and how it arouses us mentally and physically. It might be a scene from a novel or film. It might be a painting or a sculpture. It might be the forms we find in nature: how the desert scape looks like breasts and hips or how the bridge between branches of the backyard oak looks like eroticized male flesh. It might also be something much more directly erotic.

Sensuality is everywhere: in the male and female intimate shapes within flowers, in the tender and delicious food that slides down our throats, in a warm bath that makes our skin tingle, in the sand under our body on a hot summer day at the beach. Sexuality is everywhere, too: in our lover undressing next to the bed; in our partner's wet and slippery body getting out of the bath; in his morning arousal under the sheets. We can bring what turned our attention to the sensual and the sexual with us to our marriage to eroticize our body and mind when the time is right.

Let me be clear, though, I'm not talking about itching and hungering, cruising and scoping other human bodies besides our spouse's. That's a devotion issue, and it's just not honorable. Let me share a Jewish proverb that should be remembered whenever we see something erotic that we want to take delight in while still seeking to stay devoted to our partner: "God bless the world that has such beauty in it."

God bless the world that has such beauty in it gives me the opportunity to notice how the loveliness of a woman in the gym locker room putting lotion on her breasts suddenly lands on me as sensual; how the shape of a man's hips and ass as he lifts a couch onto a moving truck suddenly strikes me as incredibly masculine and strong; how the bodily press of a roomful of friends hugging upon greeting makes me feel warm and alive; how the sex scene in the novel I'm reading arouses me and fills my thoughts all day long, and then empowers my want and need for my husband on our Naked Date. That's what I'm talking about.

Thought responsibility is about using our personal sensual experiences in the world to be arousable. We've all heard that sex is thought-governed, meaning our desire comes from our head as well as our body. So we have a responsibility, I believe, to ourself and our partner, to notice what arouses us and hold it in our thoughts so we're accessible to the land of the erotic.

In other words, we have to cue our being during the day with our own imagination with what strikes us as sexy and arousing, and then savor those thoughts within the framework of a devoted marital partnership. It's about noticing what wakes us up erotically and storing it up for our partner. We need to think some sexy thoughts so we can bring them to our Naked Date, and ready our body and being to be aroused. Each of us needs to offer that.

Things strike us as sensual and sexual all the time. All we need to do is pay attention them and notice the lovely and delicious world in front of us—the blessed and exquisite experience on Earth that has such beauty in it.

Lourdes and Steve

Lourdes was raised in a very large, traditional, Mexican-American, Catholic family, which meant, in her words, "There was way too much sexual repression, and the boys got much more leeway than the girls. It infuriated me."

When she was eighteen, she moved out of the house, put herself through college, and went on what she called "a wild, sexual ride."

"I was free to do whatever I wanted to do for the first time in my life, and I did. It was a total blast."

Steve grew up in a more open, permissive family where he and his siblings were allowed to have boyfriends and girlfriends stay overnight. His parents encouraged sexual exploration by offering him explanations, books, and videos on intimate coupling.

When he was sixteen, both his parents had affairs, and then tried to have an "open marriage" for a while. "The whole 'free love' thing never appealed to me, even as a kid." Steve noted. "I always knew I wanted someone just for me, and me for her. When my parents divorced over all of it, it was like, 'Yeah, so that whole open-love thing is just messed up.' I didn't want any part of it."

When he met Lourdes, she was openly dating multiple men. "I was being honest about it—there was no cheating—but later I realized I was putting on a bit of

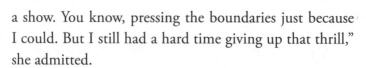

a show. You know, pressing the boundaries just because I could. But I still had a hard time giving up that thrill," she admitted.

When Lourdes and Steve began to fall in love, he gave her an ultimatum: be monogamous or he'd let her go. She agreed, and a year later they married.

In their sex life, he was more often the more reserved of the two, meaning Lourdes often initiated.

"I'd approach her too, sometimes," Steve said, "but I was much more subtle about it and she'd miss the signs."

Lourdes added, "I had this jump-on-him approach, fast and furious, like my dating life."

After a number of years, Steve began to turn off to her: "I felt like it was gangbusters sex. She came on so strong, I never got a chance to feel her or get a sensation in before she was trying to come," he said.

When we first spoke, they'd been drifting sexually for months at a time, but had still engaged in daily affection. To help them, we needed to unravel a few things. I asked Lourdes where the need to rush sexually had come from.

"I taught myself to get pleasured by a man quickly, because I never knew if the guy had the knack of a woman's body in bed, so faster was better."

"So, *uncertainty* was a sort of zero-to-one-hundred sexual aphrodisiac for you?" I asked.

"Wow. I guess so," she said. "I never thought of it that way, but, yes."

Lourdes knew that Steve needed a different pace and was more than willing to please her in bed, but uncovering the fact that a little uncertainty was a turn-on for her helped us come up with some strategies that could help get them both what they needed.

First, I invited them to try having two to three minutes of unconsummated sex play every day for a week, and I asked Lourdes not to climax at all—not even by herself—and to just enjoy getting hot.

Then I asked them to try using the Naked Date each week with one provision: they would set the timer for fifteen minutes, and I asked Lourdes to not press toward orgasm at all during that time, no matter what act they were engaged in. After a few sex encounters, they could lengthen the timer to twenty minutes, and then twenty-five. The focus we were encouraging was *sensing,* not pressing.

I also asked Lourdes not to focus on her own pleasure, but to see how Steve's body worked and to discover what she could arouse in him by trying things. (This is the opposite suggestion I've offered to women who have a hard time focusing on their own excitement and need to focus deeply on their own sensations. Lourdes was not one of these women.)

I suggested that Steve vary the routes and the ways he touched his wife's body *every time her touched her.* "Really?" he said. "That's going to take some thought."

I explained that Lourdes thrilled with a little uncertainty, and that if he wanted to captivate her and get her sexual attention, he needed to mix it up.

After trying these tips, they reported that they felt "more connected," "more explorative," and "like a light went on."

A month later, I suggested they try some accoutrements: dancing naked or half-clothed in their living room, having sex outdoors (with the thrill of getting caught not imminent but possible), play with a toy or two, spend a night out dancing at a club—anything that kept them within the bounds of monogamy and devotion but "broke the rules" a bit.

Those simple ideas opened them up to the idea of sex as play, and they started to have some genuine fun. Lourdes had a broad smile on her face when she said, "If I had known what I was missing with Steve, I would've slowed down a long time ago."

"I never thought I was the kind of guy who wanted straight, conservative sex, but I guess that's what I was putting out," Steve said.

Lourdes said, "I get it now. There's this interplay between us; he's got this teasing, sensitive thing going on, and I've got this fire and heat ready to get excited in me, and when we play back and forth with it, we've really got something mind-blowing."

"That's it," Steve said. "Temptation and teasing, fire and heat. It's incredible to have it work for us."

Don't sideline your partner

This is going to be a tricky conversation to have, but it's a much-needed one. Sidelining our partner lives in two simple arenas: 1) intrigue behavior with other people besides our spouse, and 2) scanning for and cruising other people's bodies, both in public and when we're alone.

Let's talk about intrigue behavior first, since that's the most obvious to discern.

Intrigue behavior is exactly what it sounds like: it's taking the sensual and sexual energy that belongs to our spouse and "intriguing" with another person. It's flirting with the press of intent, or pressing the boundaries of emotional and sexual affairs—even if we're not "going all the way." It's trying to get a "hit" off another human being other than our partner with the intent of juicing up our body sexually in some way.

Culturally we have had a very warped relationship to intriguing and cheating behavior. We have unclear definitions of what it is to cheat or even flirt. We sometimes justify our own behavior, while holding our partner's actions to a more devoted-and-true standard. That just won't fly to create a naked and open sex life. It absolutely will not work to create and promote passion between partners on a regular weekly basis, because we are rocking our marriage's trust.

So what's cheating? What's intrigue behavior? Here's my best definition: it is behavior that directs your sexual, emotional, or romantic energy someplace other than your spouse's direction.

Whether it's an emotional affair (an email intrigue with your old lover from college who you found on Facebook), a lunch intrigue with a coworker that never goes past hand-holding or some deep kissing, a 900-number habit, or a sex tease (half-consummated acts in the back of someone's car after work), it's just wrong. The barometer is not whether you put this sexual organ here or that organ there, or whether you used hands or mouths versus penetration, or whether you stare into other peoples' eyes just a little too long to get a sexual hit, or whether you were "just kissing"—as if that stuff is not "sexual" and somehow doesn't count because it's not full-on intercourse.

The barometer is whether you're giving your sensuality, your sexual or intrigue energy, to someone who's not your partner. That's the defining line. And if you are, you're cheating, plain and simple, and your marriage is going to suffer.

You may claim that your intrigue behavior is due to your spouse's disinterest in sex or in being close to you. But the truth is, if you're justifying in that way, you haven't had the courage to face your partner to talk about the intimate things that need talking about, or to try the things that might make a difference. You haven't had the courage you need, and you're intriguing with other people instead. You can choose that road if you want, but it leads to nothing but unhappiness, distancing, self-loathing, and misery down the road. (I can't tell you how many people I've coached who have said, "She just up and left me," but when the truth was told, they were the ones who had been flirting with others and intriguing for years, taking energy away from the marriage.)

When you do that, you're literally killing off the opportunity to bring steady and explorative intimacy into your marriage, where it belongs. Why? Because cheating or intriguing is like the wind: even if your partner pretends not to know or doesn't sense it, a reasonably awake person can always feel the wind go out of their marital sails.

Beyond intrigue with another human being, some of us like to aggressively scan and cruise for bodies when we're out and about, and that's another form of intrigue behavior. Yes, when loveliness is presented to us, we have the opportunity to notice it and say, *God bless the world that has such beauty in it.* But cruising is a destructive thing to a marriage.

You know what I'm talking about. You're out to dinner with your partner and he can't keep his attention on you because he's looking around the room for the next hot woman who comes in the door. You're trying to romance your partner over drinks but she can't stop flirting with the uber-built bartender. This is disrespectful, hurtful behavior.

If you can't keep your eyes on your loving partner when you're together, then you've got a problem. It's sidelining your partner when you do that, and it's not by any stretch of the imagination cute or fine. When a partner thinks they're entitled to that kind of cruising when they're with you—or even when they're not— you have a problem marriage on your hands, I guarantee you. You will feel sidelined and your sex life will suffer, without doubt. You will not feel respected or cherished or free to fully trust and explore.

Then there's the issue of porn. A woman friend of mine told me that her husband's porn habit on his iPad was rattling her. He travels for work two to three weeks a month, and although she's not happy about it, she's accepted that he has this "little habit." She's reluctantly grateful that he's using porn and not cheating with other women, but it still bothers her. She told me, "I go upstairs, and there's the iPad on the bed and the wadded up Kleenex in the garbage next to the nightstand, and I know he's been getting off to his porn women, and it just hurts my feelings. I mean, here at home? When I'm here? He really needs to do that?"

That speaks to a whole can of worms that nobody's dealing with in modern marriage right now. Porn is a problem not because of its explicitness, but because of its gender inequalities. Again, men are given much, much, more permission in sex and in relationships to "look" because "men are more visual than women." That's just ridiculous. There's no way to prove that assumption, and what's worse is that it's used to justify men having more sexual permission to get sexed up on other women, while women are denied it.

The simple issue with porn is this: when one standard of permissiveness and taking energy outside the marriage is offered to one partner and not the other, there are going to be hurt feelings and a sense of marginalization. That's just normal human emotion.

Then, the images of sex in porn are not just depicting naked bodies and up-close genital views—which, God knows, can be incredibly erotic. The human form in its sexuality is truly lovely, but in porn (versus sensual art) the viewing is most often populated with the kind of nonmutual sex that marginalizes women's arousal cycles—i.e., sex for men, defined by a man's visual view and his faster arousal cycles—and do not, by a long shot, depict satisfying sex for women or sex for *couples*. Site for site, I can tell you that sex for women—that is, a man pleasing a woman with prowess, control, and strength—almost does not exist. That's a huge issue. Both young men and women are being brainwashed into thinking that the skewed images of sexuality depicted in porn are how good sex is supposed to be. That leads to inept husbands and frustrated wives in adult marital sex.

That also means that the gargantuan doughnut hole of our omission to teach our teenagers the details of how to be good lovers in marriage is being filled with porn. So it's no wonder that intimacy in marriage is flailing at an astronomical rate. Sex is the glue that holds a good marriage together. Yes, communication, agreement, respect, and ethics fuel the heart of it, but it's mutually fulfilling intimacy that grants us the grace of feeling in love, year after year—and porn does not help us find that grace.

You may argue that there are sites for women—not many, but some. (If women want to look at men's bodies, they often have to look at gay male sites—a visual viewpoint that doesn't often line up with women's heterosexual desire cycles.) And, yes, women in droves are enjoying their own sexual exhibitionism by posting erotic photos of themselves on sites for viewing. No doubt it's become a more sexually permissive world where explicitness is concerned. But just like the kinds of food we put in our bodies, we have to monitor the kinds of images we put in our brains. Nonmutual, sex-for-men, no-prowess and no-mastery images are not going to help us create a sex-fulfilled love affair in our marriage.

Sometimes it is suggested—by one partner or by a therapist—that porn be shared by the couple so it doesn't live in a separate, secret life. Although this is a good thought, be careful with this. Know that given the permissiveness of our culture to look at women's bodies (for centuries men have had the buying power, so it is women's bodies, faces, and images that have been used to "sell" just about everything, including sex), we have to be careful about using porn that's skewed towards the sexual tease of women-available-for-men and offers nothing for the heterosexual woman to be aroused by.

The truth is, both men *and women* are sexualized to look at women. To see what "sexy" is by monitoring other female bodies, not by being given permission to look—up close and explicitly—at men's naked bodies. So, if you're going to share adult erotic material, make sure there's something in it for both of you.

So many women today are dealing with the issue of porn addiction and the use of marriage-marginalizing porn with their husbands, and many don't know what to do about it. Women report feeling slighted that their husbands feel allowed to take more sexual permissiveness than they're allowed; hurt that their partners are taking sexual energy out of the relationship that they'd like to have directed back into it.

And, I'll go you blow for blow that the husbands who say, "Oh, it's just fine for you, too, honey—I'm fine if you check out the hot men's bodies online," can't stand the heat in the kitchen when she actually does start to actively use porn the same way he does.

He feels compared. He feels like she's yearning for bodies better than his. He feels that it's weird that she's lusting after the bodies of young men with six-pack abs, incredible biceps, exquisitely shaped penises and asses, and may be as young as her son. He feels the wind go out of his sails intimately, as if she's taken her adoration and desire for him elsewhere. And she has. He may say he's fine with it, but he bristles every time the issue comes up, every time he barges in on her with the iPad on the bed and a bottle of lube in her hand.

That's the point. If you marginalize and sideline your partner for porn, you can expect that she or he will feel marginalized. That will make your spouse check out on you sexually faster than you can say, "Why has she shut down on me?"

Lastly, though our interior fantasy life is going to bound where it bounds, we want to try *in our behavior* to engage in sensual acts that draw us *toward* our relationship and not away from it.

Create your own erotic jungle

I want to be clear that I have no issues with naked forms or with the figures and shapes of the sex act or with viewing them. Personally, I love the forms of the erotic and enjoy viewing the human form in all its glory. In our own home, we own plenty of nude photography and paintings and have tons of erotic imagery on our walls. And that's a mutual experience for us. We choose the art, we frame it and ready it, and we put it up on the walls. That works for us. It helps to connect us to our sensual selves as we blow by each other on our way out the door.

I believe in creating what I call an "erotic jungle" in my home—a place where art, food, clothing, music, dance, and imagery conspire to help us get intimate and sexual. All of that helps us want to keep our weekly Naked Date and helps us feel like adult sexual beings so that our sensuality together thrives and we stay close in our marriage.

However, if we rely on the oftentimes non-inclusive images of screen-based sexuality offered in our culture as standard fare, we may be left out in the cold. Instead, we might have to get a little more inventive than we planned on getting. We might have to use our creativity to draw our sexuality out and not rely upon sex images that take our energy away from our marriage.

In the documentary *This Film Is Not Yet Rated*, the director and producer make the case that sex scenes in films in which a woman is receiving pleasure are most often bumped up to an "unrated" status, meaning they're branded as "dangerously" sexual, yet images of a man getting on top of a woman with no attention to her needs are

Obviously, the key in this setup was that they were both willing, and they were both finding pleasure in the act. She was willing to come back for more because she enjoyed having sex with him—not out of a sense of duty. They had tested out their scheme, and it worked for them.

That said, most of us aren't going to be able to keep up that kind of schedule even if we say we want it. It's fun to say, "Hey, let's experiment with having some kind of sex, even non-climaxing sex, for a few minutes each day for a month," and then see what happens. It's a terrific experiment in eroticism, but it takes work to create a regular, daily sexual connection. Work that can be fun for a while, but may distance us from the act because there's not enough time between sex acts to let desire build again. So we have to find our own balance, experiment with things just to see what happens, and then land on the things that help us stay open to each other.

That's where our acts of romance, kindness, teasing, affection, and unconsummated sex play can help us. When we're trying to create an atmosphere of sensuality, closeness, and play, we are helping our marriage stay close, aroused, and open. What we're looking for here is a daily connection *of some kind*. And though we may not be having sex six days a week, we are attending to our lover in some simple erotic way, day in and day out, even if it's just for a few moments, and that keeps the erotic pipes flowing freely and lushly. Then, when our Naked Date arrives, our bodies and spirits are available to love and sex, and our whole being is available for loving.

Take good care

My husband loves the movie *Diner.* In it there's a great scene in which the character Shrevie talks about sex before and after marriage. Before marriage, he says, all he thought about was sex—*can I get it, when am I going to have it, am I going to have it tonight, am I any good at it.* He wonders when he breaks up with a girl if it was because of the sex, and then he's immediately thinking he's got to find someone else to have sex with. Then he gets married and all of those thoughts and questions go away. Supposedly he can now have sex whenever he wants it, but that's not what happens. All of that accessibility leads to a whole set of new issues.

What he's alluding to is what many of us fall into in marriage. We think: *Now that I'm married, I don't have to prepare for sex anymore. It's just supposed to happen.*

That speaks to something we have to keep our finger on. That is, sex is a primitive thing. It has a Darwinian, survival-of-the-fittest spin on it, a God-given march inside us toward bonding that's very primal. It's a pheromone-friendly experience to draw another into sexual union, and we need to remain aware of that once we're in the land of domesticity.

In other words, we can't "let ourselves go" and make no effort to be attractive to our partner. Yes, we're going to age, and we're not going to have the same waistline thirty years into our marriage as we did at the beginning, but we don't want to use that as an excuse to not try to be attractive to our partner.

We want to feel pleasingly attractive as best we can. Certainly there are people who might overdo this, going to the gym three hours a day or running fifty miles at a clip in the name of fitness. We're not talking about those kinds of extremes. We're talking about doing what we need to do to feel open with our own body, for our own heart and our own partner. That might mean going out and walking for a half hour a day, taking a regular exercise class, swimming twice a week, upping the ante a bit with a weight lifting program, or whatever else works for our health and fits into our life. We want to have an ethic of doing what we can with the body we've been given so we come to our sexuality unashamed and open. This is particularly important as we age.

Weight is a huge American issue in marriage. Overeating as a source of comfort, with no care for our own appearance or how that affects our partner's ability to be attracted to us, is a deep-seated problem in our country.

I'm not saying that everyone has to be on the latest diet in order to get love. And most of us want some enjoyment out of our bodies that is not based on a perfectionist standard. We deserve that, and we deserve to be loved, too. But if unseemly weight gain is an issue, it's also an indicator that an addiction is present, and that's going to stand in the way of intimacy.

We cannot engage in food binging, overeating, careless clothing and hygiene habits, unkempt appearances and still expect our partner to feel the primitive urges we want him or her to feel in our Naked Sex. We don't have to mirror the youth-obsessed ad campaigns we're constantly barraged with. Those unrealistic standards are *not* the definition of who gets to love and be loved. But we do owe ourself and our partner the respect of presenting our being and our body as well as we can, bringing attractiveness in body, spirit, humor, love, sensuality, and appearance to our marital table, no matter our age or shape.

Put another way, we're not only taking care of our body for our own sake, we're also taking care of it for our marriage's sake—to be able to bring a sense of freedom to our intimacy that will serve our partnership over the course of years and years.

In the lovely movie *Enchanted April*, Mellersh, who has been estranged from his wife Lottie while still living with her, says a profound thing in response to her reawakening to sensuality and love with him:

Lottie: Do you think I'm attractive, Mellersh?
Mellersh: Yes, I do. One thing puzzles me though . . . why weren't you attractive sooner?

Mellersh's point to his wife is not that she suddenly needed to change bodies and be someone else, she simply needed to begin using the one she had to bring love and affection, respect and care to herself and her marriage, and when that happened it changed the whole landscape of their relationship.

Though we need to take steps to take care of ourself for the good of our partnering, it's ultimately an inside job to be attractive and to feel open with our whole being. That's our job: to do what we need to do so we can feel unashamed and free when we're being intimate with our spouse.

I like to look at it this way: my body is a gift from life itself that I offer to myself and my partner, along with a spirit of kindness and openness that I bring to my husband and my marriage. And I want to give all of it with as much love, thanks, attractiveness, and respect as I can.

Beauty in all its forms

When I lived in Los Angeles, I used to sing for a spiritual service, and I was asked to sing a duet with a terrific woman who was very different from me in shape and size. When the music director asked us to sing together, she took me aside and said, "I can't sing with you, you're too tall and thin next to me." I responded, "Sharon, sweetheart, you're just lovely, and your voice is gorgeous. Beauty in all its forms, girl." And she lit up.

That's a truism I've held to all my life. That not only do I want to see the beauty in my own form as it changes shape and ages, but I want to see the gorgeousness of other people's bodies and spirits, no matter what shape they come in—and particularly my husband's. I want to *witness* beauty the way it comes in real life—in all the exquisite and quirky and illogically lovely shapes that real human beings come in.

I practice this in the world. I look for people's beauty. And that helps me when I'm being intimate with my husband. It also lets me off the hook of perfectionism and allows me to own the good of our healthy, fleshy, warm, and lovely physical forms.

This kind of thinking is important for our self-esteem in loving. We've got to take some ownership of the beauty in our human form, and in our partner's, so we can free ourselves enough to love well. We need to grant ourself permission to revel in our own flesh.

Here's a news flash: no matter how much plastic surgery we can afford, we're all going to age. We're all going to move from the ease and grace of one era of our body's experience on Earth to another era—one that involves gravity, wrinkles, creaky joints, and more. Though we're doing our best to present ourselves in a lovely way in the world, particularly to our partner, the physical wear and tear of life is going to catch up with us and in its weird way humble us.

When my husband and I went to Venice, Italy, I had a profound experience that illustrates what I'm talking about here. As we wandered through the city, I was completely knocked out by the patinas of the homes, the rich and vibrant hues of colors on doors and walls and windows, crackled with age, everyplace I looked. But what was so astonishing was that I could see what the buildings looked like in their original form more than a thousand years ago. I could see them as young, I could see what they looked like in middle age, and that day I saw aging beauty in their cracked and patinaed hues and textures. They were like human faces and bodies.

I suddenly understood how to see my lover as beautiful his whole life long: all I have to do is look at the exquisiteness of the years etched into his face and body, just like those gorgeous walls, and I will see him for his loveliness and grace throughout time and over time.

That vision has given me a window into loving and adoring my husband *always*. I realized, looking at those artfully aged walls, that this is what *forever* looks like in a marriage: to keep looking for the beauty in my partner—physically, emotionally, spiritually, sensually, sexually, and companionably. To find exquisiteness and even splendor in both of our fleshy forms, and then draw myself into the magic kingdom of that for as many days as we're graced with life upon this planet together.

Sex over Sixty

Intimacy over sixty can go in one of two directions: 1) it can get richer, or 2) it can dry up. The difference is simple: some couples learn to adapt, and some couples don't. We want to be the kind of couples who adapt and continue loving each other as best we can. We want the joys and the glories of the richness of age, and we want our intimacy with each other to be a grace that we need not give up.

If sex has been defined by intercourse as the main dish for years and years, then when the body does what aging bodies do—i.e., it stops responding the same way it used to respond—we have to bring broader experiential recipes to our sexual kitchen.

This is where some of the things we talked about before will help. Things like having regular occurrences of brief body-to-body contact through the day, having a Naked Date that's just about being naked and holding, and having some unconsummated sex that keeps us in an aroused state. Kissing. Embracing. Lying on top of each other, fully clothed, for five minutes in the evening. Ramp-up stuff that keeps the pump primed and the body's attention to sensuality alive and well.

Then, in the sex act itself, we have to bring our inventiveness. That means we need to get better with our hands, our mouths, our accoutrements, our rhythms, our erotic play tools, and (most importantly) our expectations.

We have to work with our head. Our age is only a number, so if we're telling ourself "I'm sixty-four and I'm too old to have sex," or "I've changed too much to still be intimate," or "My equipment's not working like it used to, so I can't be a good partner," then we're letting that number govern us more than we should. We are more than a number, more than an age, and much more than the socially held (and grossly misconstrued) beliefs about what's supposed to happen at sixty-one or sixty-five or sixty-nine. We are each unique sexual beings—at every age. And we have the right to own that, to experience what's changing and how it's evolving, and to enjoy it.

Truly, there's not a huge amount of difference between being fifty-seven and sixty-three, except the faulty information that's been drilled into our heads about the numbers, but there is no ideal sexual age. There is only a journey of experience. There is no destination, no finish line to lean in to. Sure, things happen to us that we can't control, but we don't want to use age as an excuse to shut down on the very gifts that allow us to experience the grace of loving in our older years.

What we want, instead, is a wider, bigger, and broader toolbox. We want to be able to break down barriers to changing bodies by being *more* open, by getting comfortable with new rhythms, by opening up to use everything we can come up with: hands and mouths and fingers and toys—whatever we can get our hands on to play with—to stay *in* the gift of our marriage.

What we need more than anything else as we age in love is a willingness to *go slower* and play more. Everything is slower as we age. That's just what happens to human beings. So we need to adapt to that difference in pacing, to the variant experiential rhythms that come with moving into another era of life and loving.

Of course there are pills available to aid the process of intercourse in later years. If they work for you and your partner, they can be easily integrated into a Naked Date. Since you know what time you're getting together for sex and closeness, you can both plan on when the drug needs to be ingested so you're ready for your intimacy time. That's a great gift of the Naked Date—to be able to plan, arrange, and get ready.

But the key word as we age is *experimentation*. We want to be able to give up our old expectations and be willing to try new things, new patterns, new pacing and rhythms, and new ways that we can *get there*. Though we may try something that throws off our partner on a first-round lob into his or her sexual court, we don't want to let one out-of-bounds ball shut down the whole playing arena.

Think about Albert Einstein's ability to explore and experiment—or any scientist who's ever invented something. Einstein had to try different and variant themes, over and over, until he found a discovery.

If we only try something once, don't hit gold, and then say, "Oops! The test tube blew up," and then never try again, we will never get to the discovery. Remember that there was no known practical outcome for exploring space, yet our whole world has been impacted by the discoveries that resulted in robotics, battery technologies, mapping, and satellite capabilities, among many others.

That's the spirit we want to take into our loving. If what you try with your partner doesn't work at first, so what? That just means there's something else to discover, and your playfulness and willingness will aid you in the next sexual experiment.

So, press the boundaries. Vary. Try some things. Change the pace. Give up your old ways of seeing your sensual life. You never know where the path to discovery will lead.

Sex after Seventy

A friend of mine who is in her mid-seventies is dating a man in his eighties. When I asked her how it was going, she smiled and said dryly, "He's incredibly good with his hands." We laughed a lot about that, but she was speaking to an important guidepost in older loving: that is, *don't stop touching.*

As we talked a little more, she said something profound: "Older folks don't get touched. And we should be touching."

I thought about that for a long time. I realized that although our sexual desire for release is going to fluctuate, our very real *need* for human touch does not. This speaks to what we were talking about in the previous section: that sex is a journey. We have to make it our own, no matter what the era, no matter how our body is changing.

First—and this goes for lovers in their fifties and sixties, too—we need to attend to our biology. Meaning, we have to pay attention to moisture changes in intercourse. So little is taught to women and men about midlife and aging changes in women's bodies that many women are shocked to discover that they lose moisture, which impacts their enjoyment of sex. Many partners aren't aware of this challenge at all, and that can affect our Naked Date and our Naked Sex efforts, and our desire to want to have sex at all.

So we have to sort out the biological things that could get in the way of being intimate when we want to. Moisture is an easy thing to replace, so as we age we can simply adjust to this need by applying a bit of our preferred lubricating product. Organic coconut oil (which melts on contact, is safe for insertion and use in sex, and also has antimicrobial properties—something that many of the couples I interviewed reported using) can be stored in a small container in the bedside drawer and used when needed. Both partners need to be well aware of *how much* moisture is required for a mutually fulfilling experience. That means, regardless of whether we're forty, fifty, sixty-five, seventy, or older, when our bodies are changing, we've got to explore and experiment to find what works and what doesn't.

Then there's the issue of what to do. If a pharmaceutical aid is needed for intercourse or certain kinds of sexual experience, then the Naked Date helps aid the process of *when* to take a pill. That's all fine and good, but let's say the little pill brings on headaches or other side effects. Or let's say you'd like not to rely on the pill every time. Then we're back to being inventive again.

I like to think of our aging sensuality as a great sexual arc that moves us back to the things we did before we were having intercourse and relied on penetration so heavily in our sex life. In those early days of sexual awakening, we pressed, rubbed, stroked, and used our mouths and bodies and hands to get as much sensation out of each as we could. We want that ethic in our older years of Naked Sex.

There's something else. When we were young and having our first sexual experiences before intercourse, we didn't know where we were going exactly. We just had a desire to wander over our partner's skin, to discover and play and touch, to find the things that thrilled us. When we're adults, we know where all that sex play is leading, so we tend to drive our sex experiences there—to intercourse—oftentimes short-cutting the early play.

But as we age we're asked to throw out the outcome-oriented, linear direction of lots of things in life—the drive-forward press of achievement—and just allow ourself to have an experience. (This is why grandparents are so good with small children: each is very capable of magical, present-moment focus.) In other words, in our aging years, life asks us to deconstruct the lives of reaching, pressing, and accomplishment that we've led, and leads us to relish the simple gifts of being alive. That's reflected in how our sex changes over the age of seventy.

We want to be prepared for that change in body and soul. To not give up on touching and exploring because it's different, but to give in to its changing graces, to focus on the lush, the experiential. We want to allow our being to be drawn into a slower, more open-ended amorousness just for its own sake, falling in love with touching in a wholly new way by surrendering to the gifts of being alive in all its fullness and in all its simple joys.

If we see our older sexuality in that way—that it is a gift of the sweetness of being alive—then we can be freer with the changes that are happening in our body. We get to own the intense eroticism of our early sex discovery play, returned to visit us in another era, where we can throw the bonds of our expectations over the railing and sail into a new sea—one that's gliding into new yet familiar forms of heat, touch, pacing, and deliciousness, as well as a slow gratification that we had no idea was possible.

I had a friend who was guiding force in my life for many years. She used to say, "When old ways are not working, and things are moving on, you've got to say to yourself, 'Next! Next! Next!' You've got to embrace the change and trust that something *right* is coming your way."

That's what we want in our older years of Naked Sex. An anticipatory spirit of *Next! Next! Next!* that will help us draw the joys of each era of sexuality into our heart and body.

That's how we stay in, stay loving, and stay happy with the sweet gifts of arousal in our marriage for our whole life long.

Wrapping our arms around sex

We talked about the sexual and sensual things that will help us set the stage for regular and fulfilling intimacy. We talked about offering the specific loving acts that make our partner want to come back for more and help us get into our Naked Sex on a regular basis.

Here's a short and sweet list of what we came up with:

- We recognize that married love is slow to arousal, so we account for that by having a date and time for love and offer ourselves ramp-up time to prepare to get into the act.
- We recognize that we need to be arousable, so we take responsibility for getting our head and body ready for love.
- Since mutual fulfillment is our charge, we take the time to draw out our partner erotically and sexually.
- We measure arousal by matching our breath to each other, and by seeking out moisture when our partner is a woman.
- Both partners are offered physical fulfillment and release regularly.
- We use our Naked Date premise—our uninterrupted blocks of time for love—to explore, experience, and build prowess over time and over the course of our marriage.
- We develop prowess with each other's bodies by having *time-in,* week after week, using our Naked Date and the Naked Sex principles to get there.

Simply put, if we want a sensual and sexual love experience in our marriage, we have to put a bit of time and effort into it. Not a crazy amount, but enough to give both partners what they need and want. Naked Sex wires that effort into our mind, spirit, and body and brings us the joy of a terrific and sensual sex life.

For those of us who love being close to our partner, there's nothing in the world that's sweeter.

CHAPTER FOUR
NAKED AFFECTION

Be brave enough to build the intimacy you deserve

Cheryl Strayed, in one of her brilliant writings for her *Dear Sugar* column for *The Rumpus* magazine, said, "You have to be brave enough to build the intimacy you deserve."

That's a truism we're going to build upon as we talk about affection in our marriage.

Having the courage to build the intimacy we deserve means we have to stand up for it, claim it, learn new ways to express it, and then warm up to those expressions. That's certainly going to be true for affectionate touch in our marriage.

What are we really talking about when we talk about affection? We're talking about non-sexual, not-driving-toward-sex touching. This is as critical for keeping the gates open to intimacy as a Naked Date and Naked Sex are. As human beings we need the comfort, closeness, and ease in our bodies and spirits that touching brings. We need to feel *loved as well as desired*, and that's where affection comes in.

We cannot be the type of lover who only comes toward our partner for sexual contact. When we do that, we tend to press a variant of distancing behavior on our partner, essentially perpetuating a feeling that we're using him or her for a sexual high but nothing more, and that often feels marginalizing to our partner.

When we offer no comfort, no closeness, or no communion physically unless we're going to get something sexual out of it, that can seem oppressive and may put up a barrier in our partner's sensual availability. It will also block our ability to come back to our Naked Date.

If we want regular sex—Naked Sex—we also have to have regular affection. Again, this need not take a gargantuan effort. With a few simple shortcuts, we can quickly experience a big payoff in our intimate life and our availability to each other sexually.

Affection and Science

Scientists have found that just a few seconds of close, human, body-to-body contact lowers the blood pressure, lowers the heart rate, and creates measurable decreases in stress in the body.

Researchers at Carnegie Mellon University examined the effects of hugs to discern the 404 participants' likelihood to develop colds after being exposed to the common cold virus. The study found that the de-stressing effects of hugging increased the likeliness of maintaining health by 32%. Sheldon Cohen, one of the professors who conducted the study, reported that "hugging is a marker of intimacy and helps generate the feeling that others are there to help in the face of adversity." The stress-reducing benefits of hugging release a hormone in the body called oxytocin, or "the bonding hormone," which helps create attachment in relationships and also influences mood, behavior, and physiology.

In a 2011 study at the University of North Carolina School of Medicine in Chapel Hill, researchers discovered that higher oxytocin levels correlated to lower cardiovascular reactivity (e.g., lower blood pressure) and lower rates of sympathetic nervous system reactivity to stressors. (http://health.usnews.com/health-news/health-wellness/articles/2016-02-03/the-health-benefits-of-hugging)

What this means to us in our marital partnership is this: when we reach out to affectionately touch our partner, that touch creates a bond, a feeling of safety and support, with resulting positive effects on our physiology. In plain English, hugging and touching make us feel closer, better, healthier, and more bonded. That helps to support our intimate life.

Touch creates ease. That's an ethic we want with our partner. But we're in this for more than just the science. We want our partner to stay open to us on all counts, so our Naked Date, our sex life, our romance, and our affection work. We want our partner to feel happy with us, and even *adored*. And easy affection is the simplest way to express and experience that adoration.

If we want this kind of ease and grace—think lightness, joy, and good humor—we've got to offer our affection to support that.

Most of us have simple kinds of affection we engage in. But if we've let the ship slide sideways off its moorings, we might have to admit that we almost never touch our partner during the day. That's not going to work to keep intimacy, in any of its forms, alive and well.

If we haven't been touching regularly, moving toward our partner to touch can be terrifying because we may be rebuffed, pushed away, or diminished verbally in some way. It's a huge risk, and it's scary. Our partner, not used to us reaching out and solidly ensconced in his or her ice cave, is so distanced from us that one or two touches will not create an instant awakening, nor will it melt the glacier he or she has constructed for protection. Our partner may resist our early efforts, or even say something sharp, letting us know he or she doesn't trust that we will continue to be regularly affectionate. In other words—and this is true for most of us—random and intermittent affection that drops from the sky in spurts is hard to open up to and difficult to trust. So our partner may not trust our early efforts, and that can be hard to bear.

This means that when we begin, we have to bring an ethic of resilience to our efforts, as well as patience and a little bit of

Teflon—let-it-bounce-off-of-me suppleness—to being rebuffed until we both get the ball rolling in our daily touching and begin to trust it.

Now let's talk about finding the courage to do this.

When it comes to talking about or implementing delicate and difficult things in marriage, I always remember a quote that my former acting coach paraphrased from Nelson Mandela: "Courage is not the absence of fear; it's daring to do something in the presence of fear."

Having a conversation about affection, or simply reaching out to our partner for new kinds of regular touch, requires that kind of courage—the kind that's not necessarily fearless, but, as Cheryl Strayed said, invites us to begin to stand up on our wobbly legs and start to build the intimacy we want and deserve. So let's figure out how to do that.

Find agreement in your affection

Most of us did not grow up in houses populated by large amounts of physical affection. In fact, many of us never saw our parents touch each other at all. Or we may have grown up in a family that touched regularly, but also hit and slapped and verbally abused each other, so our messages about physical proximity to other human beings may have become a bit warped. We may avoid affection because we were not shown how to physically touch healthily or because physical touch also involved a violation of our personal safety and boundaries. Another possibility is that we may yearn for touch that's safe so intensely that our partner feels our need as overbearing. Any way you slice it, those of us who grew up with some version of these experiences will have issues with affection.

How do we overcome those things to get to the loving affection we so deserve in our marriage?

First, we need to be able to talk about what we need. That means— you guessed it—we have to talk about what works and try things until we find out what does. We have to give something as well as be willing to receive something, we have to listen, and we need to verbalize how we each work physically and what our needs are. For most of us, that's a little frightening.

In our first marriage, my husband and I had a very unequal relationship to touching each other, which rattled me on a daily basis. He grew up in a peaceful home in which there was steady and loyal love, but not a lot of physical affection. I grew up in a family in which there was lots of touching, but there was also plenty of trouble, anger, and mixed messages about love. My need to be touched when we were first together was huge—probably in part because I wanted my relationship to make up for the approval and closeness that I often missed growing up, and partly because I was having a hard time finding my way in the world. His need for affection had barely risen to the surface, possibly due to the fact that he wasn't used to being around someone who touched him so much, or that he hadn't ventured very deeply into the world of one-on-one relationships. That set the stage for an unequal playing out of affection, and for lots of hurt feelings and misunderstandings.

He would come home from work, enter the front door, and I would rush to him, press up against him, and passionately kiss him. I was dying to get next to him, and if I'm honest about it, I wanted his affection to make up for the horrendous time I was having in my work life. He would physically remove my hands and push my body away, saying, "Hon, hon. Okay, okay. That's enough." It made me feel horrible.

I had the sense that my husband could go for weeks and weeks without initiating touch with me, and though I knew some of that was my fault in the way I approached him, I didn't know how else to do it. I used to play a game with myself that went like this: *I will hold out from touching you as long as you can hold out from touching me.* I would refuse to initiate, and I would refuse to touch. In those days, he could literally go for weeks at a time and not come toward me. Usually, because my need was so great, I'd cave in, and the whole cycle would start again. It was deeply dissatisfying for us both.

When I think about that experience now, I realize that some of the trouble we had with touching had to do with the way I came at him, and when I played my distancing game, it gave him a break. What I also discovered when we broke up was that he secretly counted on me to come toward him—to initiate. When we were on the brink of divorce, and all of that affection had disappeared, it became very clear that he deeply missed my moving in to touch him. He wanted it.

In our second marriage, what we found by talking about that experience was that we had had no agreement about how touching worked for both of us. We were relying on assumptions that the other person's clock ticked the way ours did, and we had no ability to talk it out and figure out what might work.

Now I understand that my husband needs five minutes when he comes in the door to just settle down from his day, and he understands that I want to connect with him as soon as he's ready.

When we discussed it, we agreed that he would come and kiss me hello, then I would give him a few minutes to adjust to home life. When he was ready, he would find me and connect with me verbally and affectionately. If he forgot, I could find him and initiate. Though this seems like something we should have just known intuitively, we didn't, and it gave us trouble. With the willingness to have a specific conversation about how we're both wired in our physical needs, we were able to find a simple peace and some gratification for both of us.

That said, my husband is a lot more self-contained than I am. He can disappear into a book, a film, or a newspaper and be happy as a little clam, contented in his chair. I, on the other hand, like to be near him physically, even when we're just lying on the couch reading.

But now we understand each other's natures better. He will readily admit that he goes dark in offering affection—i.e., that it doesn't come naturally to him—particularly if he's worried or stressed. He now appreciates my efforts to touch him, and he's more receptive to them. I, on the other hand, know that when I get excited about anything in my life, I get very touchy-feely and boisterously passionate, and that

I need to measure my expressions based on what he can receive. It doesn't mean I can't be myself, it just means that I've learned to express my love for him in balance with his needs.

Since we've found that balance, he comes toward me more and more on his own, and our touching feels much more natural. When we brought a little air and breathing room into our affection—and some conscious agreement—everything became freer. That's the point of Naked Affection.

Every little bit counts

Sitting down and talking with my husband about our different affectionate natures meant we both had to implement some changes in the way we approached each other.

For me, it meant that I had to learn to use some affection strategies that allow my husband to be who he is, in his more self-contained nature, but also accommodate my need to connect. It meant I had to learn that every little bit of affection counts.

Each act of love builds upon the next, and aids both of us in feeling "in love." It doesn't have to be big and it doesn't have to be bold. In fact, often simpler is better. But I had to get used to that.

Now, when we're sitting on the couch and reading together, I may just lie sideways and put my lower legs on his lap. I may come by when he's watching something and kiss him on the head or wrap my arms around his shoulders from behind for a moment and then move on. I may press my hand to his rear end playfully in the hallway, and then let him go. Every day, I will ask him to hold me if he hasn't. In bed, if we haven't connected, I will ask to lie on his chest for five minutes, and then will let go and let him sleep.

Since I write at home, when my husband comes in he'll come over and ask me to stop for a moment and kiss me. Or he'll hold me as I'm getting dressed, or turn me around when I'm at the kitchen sink to make out with me for a minute, or just come sit by the bath when I'm in it and lean over and kiss my cheek. As I was writing this, he walked by and put his hand on the middle of my back for a few seconds, and then moved on to let me work. This works for us—to feel a more natural ease in our touching, giving him room to initiate with me while allowing me room to be who I am and have my needs met, too. It has helped to create balance, and that has enriched our entire intimate life.

In order for all of that to work, we had to talk about it. We had to try some things. We needed to allow some fresh winds to blow between us so we could experiment with some new ways of touching, and then ask for things when we needed something specific. After a short while, the asking and the implementing got less terrifying. Now it's built in to our days.

Sure, we slip into periods of drifting from each other, but when that happens I have learned to *just ask* for what I need. To say, "Hon, can you hold me on the bed for five minutes?", asking with no edge, with no anger or irritation in my heart or voice. In other words, I have learned to ask *before* I get pissed off that I'm not getting what I need. That has helped immensely to build trust in our touching.

Would I rather that he chased me all over our apartment? Some days I would, sure. Would he rather that I mysteriously drew him in from across the room instead of initiating some frisky, skin-to-skin contact with him? Sure, sometimes.

But we have also learned to accept how we're both wired and to see the good in it. To accept every little bit of touch and affectionate play as a good thing that deepens our bond, and to revere the role each of us plays in making that happen. I help us come toward each other when we're drifting; he helps us create the romantic space that allows for our desire to build. And it works.

But we didn't create that agreement overnight. We had to get divorced, be alone, get back together, remarry, and then really *work on it* before we were able to learn this.

I have an adage that I keep close at hand for these kinds of marital challenges that helps me get to the heart of things before I get angry or edgy: *What is the request behind the irritation?*

That's what we're trying to find when we're looking for agreement, or when we're looking to take the affectionate road versus the irritated one: we want to find the request that's underneath the anger and the frustration. It requires honest asking—not the pissiness, or the anger, but the *request*. We want to spit those requests out, in a loving way, as soon as we recognize what they are. And even if we don't know what they are, it's still worth discussing what they might be in an open-hearted spirit of exploration and discovery. Sometimes just by opening our mouth and rambling a bit from the heart, not the brain, we'll stumble on what's true for us.

So speak up. Find a time you can sit face-to-face on the couch and talk about how you're both wired in your need for affection. Then, with all of your fear still in your throat, touch *anyway* and make every little bit count.

Give as good as you're getting

The second thing we need to be able to get to the loving affection we so deserve in our marriage is this: we have to be willing to give as good as we're getting.

Oddly enough, this challenge is not gender-based. We often think of women as being naturally more affectionate and men as being a bit more withholding, but that's not actually true in marriage. As I found when I interviewed couples for this book, as well as in my coaching practice, human beings are all over the map in their affection needs, so we don't want to stereotype what a man should need or what a woman should give or we will unintentionally marginalize our partner. That won't work to create the personal agreement and mutuality we're seeking.

Each person is unique in his or her needs for touch and closeness, just like each partner is unique in his or her sexual wiring. When we generalize, we miss the point of reaching out altogether. Instead, we want to listen, pay attention, learn, and implement. Our goal is to find out who our partner is in relation to touch, then find a place where our personal need and our partner's nature can meet.

Simply put, affection is about making our partner feel loved. That's it in a nutshell. If we're not reaching out, if we're not touching regularly in a non-sexual way, our partner will not feel loved. Our partner may "know" that we love him or her, but he or she will not *feel* it.

Without affection, our partner may feel distant on one end of the bell curve and cold and icy on the other end, as if he or she is being treated like a piece of furniture instead of a living, breathing human being. So we have to get to our touching, even if it's imperfect.

Even more importantly, we can't have a one-sided experience in affection. If one partner is doing all the initiating, and the other partner is making next to no effort, then the initiating partner is going to feel hurt. We need to take an honest look at what we're actually offering.

Just like in foreplay, we often think we're offering much more affection than we actually are. Are we, in actual measured amounts, touching our partner affectionately at least two or three times a day for at least ten to thirty seconds? Do we have an ethic of touching as we pass each other in the house, or do we ignore each other? Do we kiss and hold and find times where we can, in a relaxed way, just have our skin touching the other person's body? Do we lie down and hold each other, even just for two or three minutes, during the week? Have we gotten lazy, allowing our partner to do all of the reaching out?

These are the questions we need to ask ourself in order to discover whether we're giving as good as we're getting. Just as in sex, we cannot set up a nonmutual experience of touching and expect to help our partner open up to love and intimacy. It just won't work.

Begin to notice how much affection you're actually offering and how much affection your partner is offering. Try to find balance. Prompt yourself to give a little more than you're giving right now, even if it's just six more seconds of contact as you're passing in the hallway.

Offer yourself to make your partner feel loved. Think about what that might be, noting how your spouse is wired affectionately. Give something that makes him or her feel adored and special. Open yourself to more closeness.

That's what we want. Closeness for the good of our affectionate experience, surely, but also because touching keeps us open to our sensuality, and all of it is good for our souls, our spirits, and our marriage.

Incremental touching

Let's say that our marriage has been drifting in its affection and we'd like to deepen our physical touching experience for the gift it will offer in helping us stay open to healthy intimacy. How can we begin? What practical steps can we take?

If we've not been touching much, we can't expect to just agree that we're going to touch and have it instantaneously work out. We've got to retrain ourselves to be affectionate, and it's best to do that in slow, steady steps.

Furthermore, one partner may have an easy time with touching based on his or her upbringing or historical experience, while the other may find it completely counterintuitive to reach out at all. That means we have to find a middle ground, and we have to approach that challenge with respect and patience.

If we've truly never had the experience of open affection, then we have to be *trained* to touch. How do we navigate those challenges as a couple?

Working with my coaching clients, I've found that the way to handle this challenge is through *incremental touching*. Here's how it works. For one month, each partner agrees to reach out twice a day with a light touch—a meaningful ten- or fifteen-second touch in a nonsexual area of the body, such as fingertips to an arm, a hand placed over a hand, or a palm held to the middle of the back. We might describe this kind of reaching out as an *innocent* touch. Every day, each spouse reaches out two times, gently bridging the gap between no touch and connecting.

Once we've got the hang of light touching, then we move to the next step: hugging. This means standing up at home or a comfortable place and hugging for ten to thirty seconds. Each spouse adds two initiated hugs to the day in addition to the light touches we've already mastered. If that feels like too much, start with one hug. The point is to slowly get used to affectionate touching. (Those of us who aren't used to hugging usually bow out after only two or three seconds, and that isn't the idea here. Stay a full ten to thirty seconds, then part gently.)

Once we've mastered the daily standing hugs, then we can add three to five minutes of body-to-body holding while lying down. Remember that what we're up to in creating affection is to have some nonsexual closeness—closeness that fuels sexual desire, surely, but that is also *separate* from it. We're after the ease of affection, and that ease will fuel every part of our marriage when we engage in it well and often.

Though this incremental and simple approach will seem burdensome and slow to partners who just want to roll around on the carpet for a half hour every day with their lover, I invite you to try it, and here's why: we're attempting to offer our less-affectionate partner a growth arc to get used to being close. It won't happen overnight, and we shouldn't expect it to. Our partner is learning, so it's important that we not press for more speed and a faster touching arc. There's a learning curve we're after *together*, and we have to give ourselves the dignity of experiencing it. So don't push, and let the exercise unfold at a pace that's comfortable for both partners.

Remember the science research from the Naked Date section? It takes between three weeks and two months to embed a new habit in our bodies and beings. So let that timeline unfold. Breathe, touch lightly, and respect the pace at which we human beings learn best.

The most important part of affection, whether with a light touch, a body-to-body hug, or deeply holding each other, is *focusing*. We don't want to be doing anything else, particularly nothing that involves a distracting device, like a phone. (Let the damn thing ring or buzz.)

We want to focus, make eye contact, and feel our partner's skin. We want to transmit love. That's what affection is all about.

Jolie and Grace

As two married women in a long-term relationship, Jolie and Grace suffered from some assumptions about how women are supposed to behave in their affection. Both were raised in heterosexual homes in which their mothers were the affectionate parent and their fathers were largely shut off from affection.

Their stereotyped assumption was that women are touchy and affection should come easily in a relationship between two women.

Jolie is a medical doctor with a vibrant family practice, and Grace is the director of a nonprofit counseling center. By the time they get home after picking up their seven-year-old son, eating, cleaning up, and then putting him to bed, they've both had full days, and they've spent a large part of the day interacting with other human beings.

"All I want when we come home is for her to *be* with me," Grace said. "To touch me or talk to me or take a walk or tell me a joke. Instead all I get is veg-woman in front of the television. I swear to God, I could just bash the thing in with a hammer sometimes."

Jolie retorted, "I'm not that bad! And I don't think it's unreasonable to want to do nothing after the day . . .

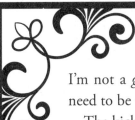

I'm not a *girl* in the way you're supposed to be. I don't need to be touching all time."

The kicker for them was that Grace had begun to turn off from Jolie sexually, feeling like the only time she was touched was when Jolie wanted some release from her. "I feel like sex has turned into a gym exercise with us, not a real connection."

Jolie felt Grace was more focused on work than on their relationship: "Why should I get up from the screen to be with her when she's got her face in her files all night?"

Grace said, "I'm only working because you're not paying any attention to me!"

I pointed out that in same-sex marriages it's important to stay away from assumptions that because both partners are the same gender they'll be wired similarly in affection, sex, and needs for closeness. That meant they had to give up the gender-stereotyped assumptions of their childhoods, and instead look across the tennis net to see who they're playing with, and then learn what works to make a match.

There was another issue: their son had recently been diagnosed with dyslexia, which meant he needed extra help each night with homework, chores, and self-care.

"I just can't do this if it's all about work and no love," Grace said. "I'm willing to try, but I'll leave if this is all there is between us."

The first thing we needed to do was help them both understand that Grace was at a breaking point and

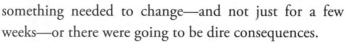

something needed to change—and not just for a few weeks—or there were going to be dire consequences.

To start, I suggested we use the light-touch idea—each partner would lightly touch the other three times a day for *at least ten seconds*, and that each would stop whatever they were doing and pay attention to the touch. To make it easier for Jolie, I asked her to count in her head ten full seconds, *one-one-thousand, two-one-thousand.*

Then Jolie admitted something profound: "I'm just not comfortable touching around our son."

I suggested that since their son has a challenge, the need for him to see and be surrounded with affection and love was even greater, and that their whole family would benefit from their efforts, however slowly the changes happened. Jolie agreed to try.

The first week the whole thing fell apart when Jolie "forgot" to touch her wife and resisted Grace's attempts to touch. I let them know that failing was part of the process and asked for Jolie's *willingness* to not only try, but to also be *giving,* meaning this effort was going to cost her something. She needed to *commit* if she wanted her married life to improve.

It worked. After they had been using light touching for a month, I asked them to progress to hugging and kissing in the house, adding one ground rule to the mix: *one hour of television or screen-focus per evening.* After dinner, Jolie got an hour to veg out, and after that, once their son was

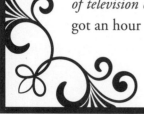

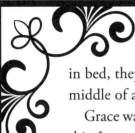

in bed, they had to turn the thing off. If they were in the middle of a movie, they'd pick it up the next night.

Grace was heartened by this idea and told Jolie, "I want this. I want to read next to you or talk or play some music and do nothing with you."

I suggested using a timer so there were no arguments about when the hour was up. When it went off, off went the screen. At first, all the couple did was read next to each other, and after a few weeks Jolie noticed that she was sleeping better. She attributed it to the "wind-down time."

Next, I suggested they try playing board games or anything that got them to focus on a bit of fun and mindlessness together. Since both women have strong problem-solving skills, board games gave their minds something to do while they playfully communicated and hung out together. Some nights they were so into it that they skipped TV or a movie altogether in favor of a game. Within a few months, the joy had returned to their love life.

"I didn't know what I was doing to myself," Jolie said. "I was wiring myself up all hours of the day, especially with what I was watching on TV. And though it hasn't been easy to start touching, I have to admit that now that we're doing it every day, it's better all the way around. Our son seems to be less reactive, and our sex is better than it's been in a long time. I just had to get it through my thick head that no one can live without love in a marriage; it has to be shown."

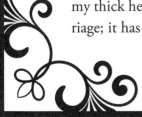

Create allure

When I looked up the definition of the word "affection," I stumbled upon the word *allure*. That sparked something important.

Affection is about much more than just getting our human need for touch met by the person who is supposed to love us. In its true, Naked Marriage-inspiring form, affection is about creating allure between two marital partners.

So, what does *allure* mean?

The American College Dictionary definition is: "To attract by the offer of some real or apparent good; to tempt by something flattering or acceptable." To be *alluring* means to be "tempting, enticing, seductive, fascinating, and charming." Well put!

Affection is more than just a biological need for human contact that we're looking to have filled, or a demonstration of safety and security that we're offering. It's about creating—just like in sex—a mutual platform of *drawing our partner out* into what is deliciously flattering, enticing, and even seductive.

To touch with the intent of being alluring means we're offering touch as a romantic act. We are playing with attraction by offering "some real or apparent good." We're tempting our partner to engage with us, moving in, pulling back, and then coming back in for a bit more—drawing our spouse into the sweetness of love.

Does that mean we have to be a virtual Don Juan or Bathsheba? No. It simply means we approach our affection with an ethic of *drawing out our partner's ardor*. That means we have to see our affectionate efforts for what they really are: an act of service to our loving.

We want to offer the exact same kinds of methods to our affection that we do with our sensual play. Again, *we are engaging in drawing out our lover*.

Living with that simple drawing out ethic is life-altering and marriage-shifting in the extreme. We stop shutting down. We start paying attention. We begin to give more. We listen. We talk. We try new things. We ask nicely. We look for things that evoke our partner's amorousness and ardor.

Marriage, as was mentioned before, is an animal that's slow to arousal. The acts of affection, romance, and love that we offer it outside the realm of our Naked Date and Naked Sex end up doing a very profound thing: they serve to fan the little flames that keep our desire and fire alive in the midst of all of the daily messes that our busy weeks serve up.

When we're willing to give and receive these little acts of love—no matter how simple or small—we tend to feel that we're living inside a romance instead of being duty-bound roommates. We tend to experience our love, rather than our obligation. We tend to stay connected, rather than drift. We have a primal, sensual experience of being in love—beyond what we may know in our head—and that makes us feel gloriously blessed, day in and day out, no matter what the week rains down on us.

Speak affectionately

Affection is also woven into the way we speak to each other. We'll talk about this more in the communication section, but it's appropriate to talk about it here, too.

Verbal affection in marriage is all about tone. If I'm honest with myself, nine-tenths of what I say to my husband is usually just fine in content, but it's my tone that's going to determine whether he gets upset with me or not; whether he chooses to be responsive or walks away in a huff.

It's easy, as we all know, to take a controlling, condescendingly parental, or slightly bitchy tone with our partner, as if we are talking to a seven-year-old child who's just not getting what we want him or her to do. This absolutely will not work to fund a loving marriage, and it also won't help us get to our intimacy each week.

We have to find a way to give up that kind of tone.

A parental tenor in our speech with our partner is an exercise in codependency—meaning, we are trying to control our spouse with shame—and if we are engaging in that on a regular basis, *we're* the one who needs help. Yes, our spouse may be inept at one thing or another—each of us usually has blind spots, failings, inabilities, and failures that impact the marriage—but if we are berating our partner for what he or she can or can't do—badgering and bullying, in the name of "guiding"—we will take all of the gas out of the hot air balloon that we're trying to fill up each week to get to our Naked Date and fuel a happy marriage.

In other words, if you talk like that to your partner on a regular basis, you will kill your sex life.

What we want, instead, is to *talk nice* to each other. Usually the reason we're unable to do that is because we have large, unaddressed, smelly, elephant-sized issues in our marriage—money pressures, debt, sexual shut-downs, or no time for each other—and instead of dealing with them, we pick on each other over little things. In the section on Naked Communication, we're going to figure out how to get those big things out of the way without burning down the house. But for now, we need to accept that we have to learn to speak kindly, with adult maturity, or we won't ever get to feel the love we have.

Once we have a communication mechanism for dealing with the things we found overwhelming—things that have been standing in the way of our love affair—we're able to feel free and open with each other again. That means we're better able to give up our mean-spirited ways of speaking. And, unless we're in a brink-of-divorce total breakdown, that kind of clear, kind, affectionate speaking tone tends to happen naturally once we have a steady framework for genuine communication, for getting the big things dealt with. When we are heard, we tend to relax, and our daily tone usually eases up.

Before we get to communication strategies in the next chapter, we want to set the stage for kindness. We want to open our mouths with sweetness. We all know that to be spoken to with ease, acceptance, and respect makes us much more willing to listen, and even more willing to learn, so we have to apply that knowledge and speak to one another affectionately.

This is another one of those realms in which I try to apply The Love Sandwich. If I have something to ask my partner or to say to him, I say something nice about him (the bottom slice), then I speak my business (the meat of the message), and then I finish with something appreciative (the top slice). Three sentences or less is my guide—two if I can manage it. Short and sweet and to the point with kindness, acceptance, and ease in my voice.

Of course, we're not going to be able to do that every time we have an issue with our spouse. Sometimes we're going to slip—we're human—and when we do, we need to apologize and change our behavior so we can better manage our upsets. Our goal is to work on the skill of speaking with kindness, and then use it *every single chance we get,* so we preserve our ability to be intimate and affectionate with each other. When we can't control ourself verbally with our partner, we ding our affectionate life and shut it down, which can also take out our sex life. Who wants to be close to a partner who's always blaring at us?

Lastly—and this relates very directly to having affectionate ways of speaking to one another—it's terrific to have some pet names. I go through phases with this: Darling, Gorgeous, Lover, Babe, Honey—it doesn't really matter, as long as I'm offering my lover some indication of who he is to me, especially when I'm asking something of him. My husband has a special pet name that he uses for me, and the minute he speaks it, I'm reminded that he adores and loves me.

Just like our romantic gestures, these classic ways of addressing each other work well because we know what they mean. They are shortcuts to softening the other person's heart. That's what we're talking about when we say we want to speak affectionately: we want to use every-thing we can get our hands on verbally, in both our words and our tone, as often as possible, to speak to our partner with loving affection.

Manjula and Ramesh

Since Manjula and Ramesh's families are originally from India, their challenges with affection were wrapped up in some cultural barriers that were barring them from having the modern marriage they wanted.

They met working as computer programmers at a large technology firm in California, and though they were both brought up in relatively progressive households in this country—Ramesh since he was five, and Manjula since her elementary school years—they both carried the weight of gender and cultural expectations from their heritage.

Their challenge had to do with a lack of touch and easy access to affection in their marriage.

Manjula is incredibly gifted at mathematics and excels in her work, which she felt had influenced her ability to be physically available. "I work in this highly mathematical man's world, and I suppose I am used to this distance between me and men," she explained. "Between that and the traditions I was raised with in our community, I guess I'm not very affectionate."

Bucking his heritage's tradition, which prohibits kissing in public, even between married partners, Ramesh was yearning for a more open experience with his wife. "It's ridiculous," he said. "We weren't raised in India, our parents aren't around us most days, and they're not really offended when we're affectionate, anyway. We're married! Why shouldn't we be able to touch each other?"

When we discussed the issue a little more, Ramesh confessed, "I'm terribly unhappy right now. I love this woman, but I'm an American. I want to behave like one—to go to the movies and put my arm around her or kiss in her in the street if I want to. Even at home she's like this. I don't want to be strung up by these old traditions that don't help me feel my love for her."

They both agreed that they had no philosophical or religious issues with having "a modern, American marriage" where touch was concerned. In practice, though, they had not been able to bridge the idea of a close, affectionate experience with their daily actions, which meant we needed a *practical* approach.

Interestingly, the affection issue had not stopped them from being sexual regularly, but the separation between sex and "regular life touching" was rattling Ramesh so much that he felt immediately hurt after intimacy by "having my wife go cold on me the minute we stand up from the bed."

Very calmly, Manjula said, "It's not that I'm opposed to open affection. It's just that I don't even know if I can *think* that way. I'm so unschooled."

Her comment provided the opening to the practical strategies I could offer them. Our objective: *school them both* in the affectionate actions that each could offer, accept, and feel fulfilled by, a little at a time.

While they began to implement strategies, I asked Ramesh to be patient while Manjula learned—recognizing that she was willing to learn—and to acknowledge everything she did that was affectionate, no matter how small.

Manjula was willing to try because she saw how deeply her husband's unhappiness was affecting them both.

I asked Manjula to first implement a "light touch" approach: to find exactly two moments in the day that she could offer a light touch to her husband, but it needed to be a meaningful touch, not a brushing-by experience. For example, if she was going to touch his arm with her fingertips, she would stand still and engage in that touch for at least ten seconds, and, if possible, look into his eyes while touching him. If she was going to put her hands on his shoulders from behind while he was seated, she might say something nice to him.

I gave the same instruction to Ramesh, asking him to not push farther than light touching, two times a day, and with a meaningful ten-second pause, so that each partner could focus on the touching and the sensing.

"I don't know if that's going to be enough for me," Ramesh confessed. "I feel like I'm starving for her affection." However, he agreed to try.

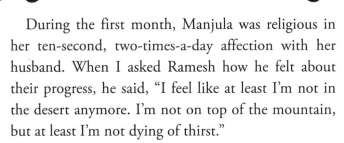

During the first month, Manjula was religious in her ten-second, two-times-a-day affection with her husband. When I asked Ramesh how he felt about their progress, he said, "I feel like at least I'm not in the desert anymore. I'm not on top of the mountain, but at least I'm not dying of thirst."

We upped the stakes for the next month, adding ten seconds of holding each other—hugging—standing up someplace in their home, and two acts of hand-holding in public on the weekends or any other time when they were together all day. After a few weeks, we met for a check-in and Ramesh said, "When I reach out to her and she doesn't avoid me or push me away, that's when I know this is working."

At month three we upped the stakes again, working up to what I call "sweet kissing" in public: a little longer than a greeting kiss, but not so long to embarrass Manjula. It worked.

By the time we added five minutes of nonsexual holding on the bed or couch each day, the ice had melted between them, Ramesh's irritation had faded, and Manjula had become more comfortable with touching her husband.

"I think I had this stereotype in my head that touch was supposed to be initiated by my husband, but only in limited, very private moments, and I didn't realize how powerful it was to draw him to me with it. To

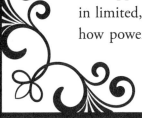

see him light up when I reach to hug or touch him has altered me so much. It's made me more available to initiation in our lovemaking, too, and that's been a wonderful turn for us."

Ramesh agreed. "I'm more at ease with her, and I'm not counting the times she pulls away and keeping score like I was before. . . . She made this effort for me, to be closer to me, and it makes me very emotional when I think about it. I feel like she's *with me* now."

When the roof caves in

Many of us are actually pretty good at being affectionate and kind to our partner, both verbally and in our behavior, a lot of the time. Where we go awry is when something unpleasant happens. We may use these experiences as an excuse to go ballistic, or to deteriorate into crazy worry and obsession, barraging our partner with all of that intense energy.

Marriage does not withstand that stuff well. Even though our partner is our closest ally, and he or she is the person we will need to share most things with—particularly things that affect our life together—we have to be better and stronger than dumping our angst upon our spouse.

Our partnership is a delicate balance. Though we don't want to ignore large problems, we also don't want to catastrophize in spirit or in action. When we catastrophize, our spouse feels it energetically as a commentary on his or her ability to take care of us, to help keep things going smoothly. It's a type of criticism: that he or she couldn't keep the ship sailing straight for us. It shuts off our partner's affectionate, sensual, and romantic feelings, as well as our ability to problem-solve as a team.

Know that the only options the observing partner has during a spousal freak-out is to try to tamp it down or to retreat.

Either way, when we erupt, the issues get sidestepped, and we end up using our partner as a counselor for crisis intervention. That won't work.

There's another aspect of this that's worth mentioning. When we disintegrate into a worried, obsessed mess, or we "lose it" in frustration—even if the eruption is about something not related to our couple experience—it doesn't give room for our partner to have feelings. If we're always blustering and bellowing when something goes wrong, or spewing when we're frustrated, our partner will learn not to trust us with intimate feelings in order to guard against our next blowup.

There's no room for both partners when one of us has complete control of the game board with a messy emotional eruption. That won't help to create affection or trust, and it won't help us get to our weekly Naked Date, or romance and sex.

If we've been blasted by our spouse's waiting-for-the-next-shoe-to-drop emotional time bombs, there's no way we're going to want to get next to him or her naked. It's too scary, and makes us too vulnerable. Nine times out of ten, when there's an unequal blasting of the room from one partner, the other partner will just shut down—sexually, emotionally, and spiritually.

So we have to give up those blaring, down-the-rabbit-hole expressions of emotion and develop some chops for problem-solving as a couple. We have to apply our resilience, our patience, and some emotional self-control for the good of our affectionate bond.

Our partner is not our therapist. He or she is not a best friend with whom we can dish any dirt we choose to dish. That's not the nature of our relationship. It's much more frail and interdependent than that. To put it bluntly, marriage does not do *venting* well.

If we need the kind of support that allows us to just vent our feelings and have someone hear our eruptions and our head-spinning worries, then we need a therapist, a clergy member, a trusted friend, or a support group (Co-dependents Anonymous or Al-Anon Family Groups, for instance) where we can take our volatile emotions and process them.

We cannot—repeat, *cannot*—take those emotions to our marriage and expect to have consistent intimacy between the eruptions, obsessions or spun-on-its-head worry. It's just not going to occur. Blowing up or falling apart on a regular basis is a selfish mechanism used to control the room, to shut everyone else up, to badger and bully our partner into quietude—whether directly or passive-aggressively—so we don't have to deal with his or her opinions or feelings and can splatter the room with our own. We are literally consuming all of the space for feelings and emoting when we do that, and our partner will almost always shut down on us, particularly intimately, because of it.

Even if the issues we're tripping over are not couple-focused—i.e., if the blowups are about our own inability to find work we love or our difficulties getting along with an unreasonable boss—it's still not okay to bring that crap home and dump it into our lover's lap.

What we want is a partnership that can withstand trouble, *yet still be affectionate and kind.* We can't kill off the willingness of our partner to stay affectionate with us through life's troubles by behaving badly. And make no mistake about it, badgering, blustering, blow-hard eruptions, falling apart, and obsessive worrying are all bad behaviors. We're adults. That means when we need help, we have to go get it. We don't get to dump our troubles on our marriage.

Just like in our Naked Date, where we're trying to get to our loving no matter what else is going on in our week, we want to be able to be kind, level-headed, and physically loving to each other even when the roof caves in. And guess what, roofs cave in. That's life. Stuff shows up. Things fall apart. So if we're constantly rocking the boat of our marriage's serenity with our outbursts—killing affection in its tracks—then we need to get some help with anger, with how to manage frustration, and with how to weather trouble without falling apart. That help needs to come from someone other than our spouse or we're going to rattle our partner so severely that we'll block every loving expression in our marriage, now and forever.

An affectionate tone at home

In my own marriage, I've had to learn this the hard way. I'm usually pretty even in my emotional responses, but the thing that can set me off is having my home-based technology—which I rely on very heavily to work—fail on me, as it regularly does. Since I'm no expert at troubleshooting, I have often blown up at my computer within my husband's earshot, swearing, cursing, and promising to throw the damned thing right out the window just to watch it crash.

After a while, my husband asked me to either get a new computer and get some help with using it, or learn to take those emotions somewhere out of his earshot. It was some work for me to do that, but

I understood that what he was asking for was more than just easy communication and a spirit of affection between the two of us: it was even-toned peace and kindness *in our house* that he wanted, no matter where the energy was directed. It was rattling him to have me yell and curse like that, so I had to adjust for the good of our home life.

That doesn't mean the two of us don't get upset once in a while; of course we do. But that's not the norm, and it's not the tone in our home.

Expecting our partner to "just take it" because we're upset is not a mature stance in loving. It's not mutual, and it's not respectful. Instead, we want to speak to each other with affection, respect, and evenness in our tone. We want access to our marital problem-solving skills, while keeping hold of an ability to speak evenly and reassuringly to each other, and to be affectionate in both our physical touch and our verbal kindness.

That's what's going to support the goodness of our bond, the sweetness of living together, and the commitment, over weeks and weeks, to keep being regularly intimate with each other. It's an entwined circle: assuring, affectionate touch and speaking affectionately helps lead us back to intimacy and sex, and regular and fulfilling sensuality tends to ease everything and make life more livable.

Giving is different than generosity

Being generous and being giving are two different things in marriage. Generosity is essentially sharing. It's, "I have lots of this stuff, so why don't you have some." Generosity comes easily. It's based on contributing or gifting something which comes naturally to us.

Giving, though, is a whole 'nother animal. Giving is an act of effort that asks something of the giver. Put a different way, *it costs the giver something to give what he or she is giving*. It involves effort, and it's important to understand this distinction when we're learning how to offer our affection in marriage.

So much of how we approach marriage in our cultural timeline is based on an assumption of naturalness, meaning we have been led to believe that marital communion should "just happen." We think that because we were once naturally simpatico, we should not have to make an effort to find our way to closeness later on. We tend to measure every experience of our marital lives by the small window of time when we were falling in love together, and then we're disappointed that the automatic dovetailing of energy that happened then hasn't continued through years of being together.

One of the reasons for this division in our hearts is our lack of understanding of the difference between generosity and giving. Simply put, for a happy marriage to occur over time, giving must be at the center of it. Not just the generosity of our early moments of dating, or the ease of offering things that come to us naturally—but actual, adult *giving*.

What does that mean in practical terms?

It means that we have to be able to *hear* requests from our partner, take them in and value them, and then work—sometimes hard—on offering what he or she wants from us, *even when it costs us something*.

I once had a very frank conversation with my dad about this, which clarified the exact nature of what I'm talking about here. I was talking to him about rekindling my relationship with my husband, and I mentioned that it was hard for my husband to be affectionate with me on a regular basis, particularly after being single for a long time. I said I hated always having to ask, but I knew it was better that I did, and that we were relearning how to be with each other, how to find out what worked.

My dad said, "That's good. Because that's something that I screwed up with your mother before we got divorced. If she asked me for something, I felt like I shouldn't give it because then she would think I was doing it just because she asked and not because I wanted to. And that was stupid."

My dad's error speaks to our skewed thought processes about giving in love. Lots of us have the same thought my dad did: if our partner asks us for something, we will somehow allow ourself to be controlled by "giving in" to the request, so we resist giving it. Or, worse, we tell our partner (or insinuate) that he or she is off-base, crazy, or wrong for wanting what he or she has asked for.

When we engage in that kind of resistance, we train our partner to have no needs. We block his or her ability to be allowed to want things and to have those wishes fulfilled. If he or she cannot ask and be heard and responded to, then we are obstructing the very communication that would allow for a pathway to more satisfaction, more happiness in the relationship. We are blocking ease and contentment, and we are forcing our partner into a corner. To have their needs met, our partner may passive-aggressively hint; throw a fit (which usually won't work either); or give up on having needs altogether, living in dissatisfaction.

None of that works to keep a marriage healthy. It's not a big stretch to figure out why. In a resistance setup, there's no openness, no flow between partners, and no willingness. Over time, a marriage will slowly begin to erode and fall apart with that kind of holding out. And, why wouldn't it? One partner's needs have been relegated to the dark corner of the basement, and we have instead a freeze-out of any mutual communication, needs fulfillment, or expressions of wants at all. There is no pliability, no open exploration, and no humility. None of that will build an affectionate, happy love affair.

That's not to say that every request—for affection or for anything else—will always be a "yes" or a jump-to-it effort on our part. We do have the right to say "no" to requests, but in our loving, most often, we want a spirit of saying "yes," and really *meaning* it. In other words, we're able to grant the request with genuine effort.

Lisa and Finn

Lisa and Finn met on a whirlwind vacation in Europe in their late-twenties. After talking to him in a gift shop, they went to a café and talked for hours. Lisa discovered Finn had been raised in the same city she was, where she still lived. They ended up having a romantic and steamy two weeks together, having tons of great sex, seeing the sights, and touching and holding each other all day long wherever they went.

"It was a total turn-on," Lisa said. "All of that instant love affair stuff you read about but never believe happens, that was those two weeks. I loved it."

Finn said, "That kind of thing had never happened to me, and I just went for it."

Once they were back home, they started a long-distance relationship going back and forth from Finn's place in New Mexico to Lisa's in Northern California. They saw each other every three or four weeks for a few days, and it was always a very passionate reunion, with lots of touch and intimacy, fueled by longing and hour-long phone calls in-between their weekends together.

A year later they got married, and Finn moved back to Lisa's city.

"I had to remake myself," Finn noted. "I was moving for her, for us, and since I have a referral-based business, I had to start all over. It was hard."

"I felt like once he moved in here his focus was all over the place and not on us; it was a letdown," Lisa said. "We're not kids, so I don't know what I thought I was getting into—I mean, the real world will encroach upon you for sure in a relationship, but I guess I expected more"

They had a baby in their first year of marriage, a little boy, and though Lisa thought that might satisfy some of her needs for affection, it didn't. "I love my son, and he's a little ball of joy for me, but I want my husband, too," she said.

"The problem is I feel like she's always wanting more," Finn explained, "like I'm supposed to keep up that passion we had in Europe all the time, and I can't do it."

Lisa said, "I guess I do kind of want that. I feel bummed out that that's gone."

By the time we spoke, three years into their marriage, a destructive dynamic had set in. Lisa would come up to Finn and try to kiss him or press against him, and he would push her away. "He slithers out of the way like a snake, like he can't wait to get away from me," she said. "I get really hurt when that happens, and it happens a lot, and then I get pissed off and angry and I snap at him. And who wants to touch someone who's snipping at them? I wouldn't."

Because their issues with touch weren't about enjoyment—Finn admitted he loved touching his wife—but about *approach,* we needed to use some practical strategies to improve their situation. They also needed to be easy to apply, so the tension in their marriage could be eased quickly.

I offered what I knew from a similar experience in my marriage—that the less openly affectionate partner (in this case, Finn) needed to be given some room to find his own way to his partner. However, we also needed to set up some bottom-line expectations so some of Lisa's needs could be met. Since their affection issues had impacted their ability to be sexual regularly, we needed to address that as well.

We began with the incremental touching strategies, month by month, and we added a buffer of time when Finn comes home.

Since Finn is a chiropractor, and has his hands on people all day, he needed a bit of time when he came home to relax and de-stress before engaging in his wife's need to touch. Lisa agreed that she'd be happy if Finn would kiss her meaningfully at the door when he came in, and then she would allow him some space to sit for ten minutes with their son, which he loved to do at the end of the day.

After ten minutes she could find him and they would then talk about their days, and then get up and hug each other for at least ten to thirty seconds. I

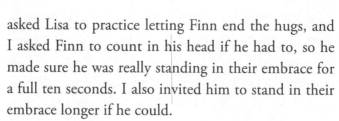

asked Lisa to practice letting Finn end the hugs, and I asked Finn to count in his head if he had to, so he made sure he was really standing in their embrace for a full ten seconds. I also invited him to stand in their embrace longer if he could.

Lisa voiced her concern, "You're kidding me, right? I'm supposed to be satisfied with ten seconds a day?"

I reiterated that we were going to apply the light touch, standing hugs, and body-to-body holding approaches, too, month by month, but in increments. Lisa was doubtful. "I just don't think having him touch my arm is going to make up for what I'm not getting here. I want him to want me. Is that so wrong?"

I asked her to be patient and to do the exercises like a science experiment, just to see what would happen.

After the first month, she reported being surprised by how little it took to make her feel loved by her husband. "Anything he does to initiate makes me feel good. And even though this ten-second thing feels like a lot less than I want, it's sort of incredible. I just warm up whenever he comes toward me."

Finn said, "I guess I need a little room—more than she does. But we got into this bad dynamic when I moved here and I wasn't paying much attention to her. . . . She probably was feeling like, 'Hey, why'd this guy marry me if he was just going to ignore me?' So,

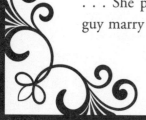

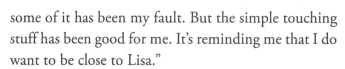

some of it has been my fault. But the simple touching stuff has been good for me. It's reminding me that I do want to be close to Lisa."

In month two, Finn said he missed being sexual and felt ready to start practicing the Naked Date. I encouraged them to not expect perfection the first month out—with either the incremental affection strategies or the Naked Date attempts—to give themselves some time to try and retry until the strategies made a difference. I specifically invited Lisa to let their relationship be "imperfect" for a time while they learned this new way of being close.

The Naked Date worked very quickly for them to restore their sexual connection, and, because it was an every-week event, it made Lisa less resistant to the daily ten- to thirty-second affection efforts they were making, which also made Finn more willing to use them.

Four months later, they both agreed that they were "out of the woods." Finn said, "The thing is, we never stopped loving each other, we just needed some help getting through a big misunderstanding. That's what it feels like to me."

Lisa said, "This whole thing was good for me, though I wouldn't want to revisit the pain. I needed to calm down a little about my need to touch him, and when I did I got him back, and now I feel like it's better than ever."

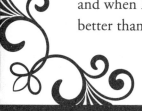

The real world of affectionate giving

So, how do we manage this in the real world? What happens when we're asked for something from our spouse and it's hard for us to give it? When it doesn't come naturally, how do we offer our efforts with any hope of satisfying our partner?

Here's where the magic of giving comes in. When our spouse asks us for something that's hard for us to give, and we work with diligence to give what was asked for, our partner notices the effort and is heartened. Meaning that even if the giving is imperfect, our spouse will appreciate the lengths we go to. Our partner notices that his or her request *mattered to us*, and in turn knows that he or she matters because we paid attention, and then tried our best to offer what was asked for. That's huge.

The next time *we* ask for something, our spouse will remember the efforts we made, and he or she will be more willing to give to us. Our loving and our offering then becomes this beautiful figure-eight of you give to me, then I give to you—a demonstrated willingness with each other that builds a solid, flowing foundation of love. That willingness builds trust and freedom, as well as more love and happiness.

Though this ethic of giving versus generosity applies to almost every topic in this book, I'm talking about it here because open and regular affection usually requires effort for both partners. It asks that we move beyond our comfort zone, as well as our day-in, day-out unconscious distancing behavior, for the good of our marriage. And it asks that we do it again and again, not just for a week or two. Most of us are going to have to practice, fall down, and then get up again and practice some more before we get this. We are going to have to work to discover the land of giving in physical affection—the kind *that meets our spouse's needs and even exceeds them*—in every affectionate effort we make.

In my own marriage, when we finally learned how the generosity-giving continuum worked between us, it literally changed the landscape of our whole loving experience for the better. Everything in our life together changed once we became willing to listen, act, and work on giving to each other.

Let me offer a practical example of giving-versus-generosity from my own life. I know that my husband is excellent at buying little gifts. Many times, for no reason, I'll come home to a small, artsy present he found or a single, exquisite rose he bought to brighten my day. He's great at this, and he does it often. It comes to him naturally, and I appreciate it. I love it.

As for me, I'm a terrific home chef, so I offer my husband exquisite meals several times each week. He often jokes about it to his male friends who come over for dinner from time to time. "Yeah, guys. I *do* eat like this every week," he'll say, smiling. He always thanks me after I cook, and I'm grateful that he notices and enjoys my efforts. Both of these things live in the realm of generosity for us, and they are efforts that come easily to us—things we would still do even without each other.

Our giving lives in another category, and our affection is a great example of how this has played out. When we're busy or stressed, my husband tends to go dark on offering hugging and kissing and I have to ask for it. When I notice us drifting like that, I have learned to ask for affection in a sweet voice with "I" messages. For example, "Honey, can I ask for something? I feel like we've been drifting and I could use some more affection. Can we hold and kiss a little more?" And he will say, "Sure."

There's no judgment, no angst, no blame from me, just a *request*. But the key is that he doesn't blow me off. He listens and makes the honest effort. And I thank him for his efforts.

The same has been true for me. When I'm deep in my writing or book marketing, I tend to dissolve into talking to him with my face in the keyboard, not really paying attention to him. He will sometimes say, "Hon. Would you mind closing the computer so I can talk to you?" That wakes me up. I'll take a few minutes to wrap up what I'm doing, then power down the computer, and pay some attention to him. And it works. I listen, I'm willing to notice when I'm getting out of balance, and then attempt to balance my needs with the needs of our marriage.

There are bigger quests that have required me to learn the giving-versus-generosity continuum as well. When my husband and I first got back together, I realized that I was going to cause real damage to our marriage if I kept doing work that I hated. For the good of our partnership—and for my own ability to bring kindness and ease to it instead of angst and agitation—I had to give up the bigger paycheck and make the effort to find something else to do for work that wasn't causing me grief. It was one of the most difficult things I've done in my life, and I did it as an act of giving—to myself and to my marriage. It was a gigantic change for me, truly. It cost me my "important" career identity, and made me get honest about what might be a humbler career choice, but would bring more happiness to my own heart as well as our marital life.

The kicker was that when I got the humbler job—writing books and teaching yoga versus the intense pressure of fundraising—I was able to be more creative and loved my life ten times more. My relationship's needs ended up guiding me to what was best for me, too, and I was deeply appreciative to my husband for the impetus to make a happier choice.

That's what affectionate giving looks like. It's work, without doubt, but it's good work: honorable-and-true efforts that make loving and partnering happier, deeper, and sweeter.

Surely, every act of giving could be qualified as an act of affection. Whenever we offer our labor and our energy to change something for the good of our marriage, we are engaging in an affectionate act. We are saying, "You are worth it to me to work on this, and I see that our relationship will grow and be happier if I try to do this, even if I do it imperfectly."

That's the spirit we want to take into our affection—both our literal touching and our willingness to make efforts for each other. This spirit will bring peace, ease, grace, closeness, and a free-flowing affection into the daily experience of being together.

CHAPTER FIVE
NAKED COMMUNICATION

Communication fuels sex and intimacy

Naked Marriage, in its simplest form, encompasses the idea of regular, set-aside time for the things that support intimacy. That includes time for romance and desire ramp-up, affection and play, sensual exploration, and straight-up sex. But philosophically, it's much more than that. It's a principle we can use to guide our marriage, a concept of loving that invites us to consciously make time for the things that are really important in our partnership, particularly the things that can get bowled over in a busy life.

In its broader concept, being "naked" is about being transparent and honest and available to each other. That means the naked idea can help us in other areas of marriage, which help keep our connection strong. The big two are: communication and money. Why do we need to talk about communication and money in a book about intimacy? Because when there's trouble with either of these things, *it will block our path to the bedroom.*

In this section we're going to talk about simple, easy strategies for checking in with each other. If we want to have a loving, sensual connection, then we have to have some way to communicate about the big things in marriage. Put a different way, we need to be able to talk to each other about the things we need and want, how we choose to live, our children and our adult parents, our money choices, and more.

When we think about intimacy, we usually associate it with sex. But intimacy is a much broader experience. It's the ability to know each other, to discover more together as we live, to find shared values with the things that make life peaceful and happy.

Marriage, beyond falling in love, is about building a path with each other for a whole and contented life. When we make the effort to do that in the arenas beyond sexuality and romance, it tends to make the sex flow, too. It becomes worth the effort to us because it will lead us back to being skin-to-skin together with no obstacles in the way.

The reverse is also true. When we have breakdowns in communication, arguments about our ability to pay attention to our marriage, unaddressed money pressures, unspoken resentments, or a dreaded sense that it's no use to bring issues up, we end up feeling beaten down, and that tends to ding and drain our sex life. We cannot come to each other unburdened, so we often stop moving toward each other altogether. Our blocked communication ends up blocking our ability to be sensual as well.

The truth is, it is almost impossible to have any kind of fulfilling, regular intimate life when we are not communicating well. Sensuality requires vulnerability, and we can't be vulnerable if we're pissed off at each other and can't talk about it or are in a silent standoff. Sure, we can blast through to edgy, angry sex once in a while when we're fighting or distancing, but if we want to have a loving and sexual partnership *over time*, then we have to attend to the things that get in the way of the flow of intimacy. The most important of these, without doubt, is communication.

I used to have this entirely backwards. When I was dating, I would try to press for a sexual connection right off the bat to see if a relationship would work. I had all of my eggs in the *cha-cha-cha* basket. But without stopping long enough to notice whether or not I could communicate with a partner, or if my values lined up with his, I was putting the cart before the horse, which meant that the sexual experiences often burned out quickly and I found myself looking across the table at someone I wasn't sure I even liked, let alone had the capacity to build something long term with. I thought sex was the impetus, and if I got that right, then everything else would fall into place. But it didn't.

I had to learn that sex and intimacy are the *out-picturing* of our how well our agreement is working as a couple and not vice versa.

In marriage, we can't assume that we can barrel through all of life's challenges by jumping into bed. This is tricky to say, because sometimes we can solve a few things with a good romp. When we need to calmly agree to disagree on something, sex can be the cement that allows us to stay close while still offering each other room to do things differently in the world. Put another way, intimacy can help us stay dear to each other even when there's an upset that we can't solve.

But sex as glue will work from time to time *only* if there is an overall solid agreement between us about the basics in life: lifestyle, values, time, money, where to put our efforts, how to raise our kids, and how to talk about all of it. We need to know what we're building in the world together, and be at least somewhat on the same page with those goals, even if each individual partner is having different experiences and developing different skills sets. And the way we find this agreement is—you guessed it—through *communication*.

That means we have to talk. Not just skirt around stuff, not just make assumptions, and not glaze over things. We need to sit down, face to face, apart from all of the distractions of life, and *talk* and *listen* to each other. That's the only way we can create agreement and peace in our marriage.

That peace is the exact bedrock we need to fund an intimate life. There is no other way to build our castle together, with both of us fully invested in its construction, and still stay open to each other sexually. I'm going to say that again: *There is no other way to find the*

agreement that builds intimacy besides sitting down, and then talking and
listening to each other.

Why do we care if we're both fully invested in the actions of our
life together, in the things we do as a married couple? Because when
we're not both in on the decisions we make, we tend to marginalize one partner's input, sideline it, or ignore it, and that throws up
roadblocks between us, cutting off the road to intimacy. Intimacy is
a delicate object: it requires an even, equal flow of participation, a
mutuality of giving and receiving. It relies on more than just touching.
It's a dance of sharing, speaking up, affection, agreement, decisions,
and experiences—both internal and external—and it balances itself so
very gently from day to day.

Inclusion of both marital partners' needs, thoughts, concerns, and
wants is a big deal, and we need to find a way to get to that kind of
listening and sharing if we want a healthy intimate life.

Short and Sweet

While I was writing this book, I researched dozens of relationship and
marriage books, and almost all of them focus heavily on communication skills. But many of the strategies offered felt cumbersome and
overdone—too time-consuming or impractical to manage in a busy
married life.

Some invited my husband and me to do an archeological dig into
our marital past to dredge up old hurts so we could "see the path of
our marriage." Some asked us to engage in long, drawn-out "connecting" experiences, many of which took weeks or months to complete.
Some proposed approaches that included lots of journaling and note-
taking on the things that work and don't work. Some suggested spending weeks researching our partner's childhood experiences.

Though I believe that all of these strategies have some merit,
I often came away from these books thinking that the ideas were
too time-consuming for those of us who are basically okay in our

marriages, but who want to enhance our loving. Many books were also too focused, for my taste, on a past we had already weathered. If I'm honest, many of them made me feel like, *Yeah, we're never going to do that.*

I absolutely believe that good communication is the bedrock of a working marriage, but I need the strategies to be short and sweet—shortcuts that are applicable in the real world. I need to have a way to check in with my spouse that doesn't consume our life, and that works when there's trouble as well as when we just need to express how we're each doing.

Don't get me wrong. I'm not saying that if there's a huge elephant in the room that's never been dealt with that couples should overlook it or pretend it's not there. For instance, if one partner has been cheating for years and the other is ignoring it, that's worth a face-the-music dig into what's been happening and a request to stop it. It's also worth the effort to find a way to heal the sex addiction of repeated cheating, and then try to rebuild the marriage if that's possible. That will be a huge effort, and it will take some real digging, healing, reconnecting, and a lot of time-in. In-depth strategies, like the ones in some of the books I read, are needed in this instance, along with therapy, guidance, and slow, intricate steps.

But as I said, *Naked Marriage* is not a book for couples who are in dire straits, are on the brink of divorce, or who need some serious intervention to have a glimmer of hope of moving on together. This is a book for people who know they love each other, but need some simple strategies to get to the love they know they have.

That includes our communication strategies. We don't want our mechanisms for talking to each other to be so cumbersome that we try them once or twice, and then stop altogether, or find that we resist doing them at all. We want simple, easy, workable ways to check in, listen, speak up, and hear one another. We want to be able to move swiftly and smoothly from listening to giving.

One part speaking up, one part listening

What simple strategies can we use to get our marriage to a place of regular listening, sharing, and giving? First off, we need to talk about what communication is. So many of us have been bullied into believing that talking with our partner means fielding bombastic rants or pent-up accusations, or having to put up with being a dartboard in an angry, one-way conversation. These kinds of set-ups will not work to fund a healthy flow of marital back-and-forth. We have to find a way in which the true experience of communication can occur.

In its simplest definition, communication is one part speaking up, one part listening, and one part accommodating and adjusting. That's what's going to make this talking-to-each-other thing fly.

Think of it this way: there are three entities in your partnership—you, your spouse, and the marriage itself. Three very distinct personalities, each with needs, wants, concerns, and desires. Each needs to be fed and nurtured, listened to and attended to.

When we talk about communication, ultimately we're talking about finding acceptance and agreement, but not always at the beginning of a discussion. A lot of times what we need to do is clue our partner in about where we are—in our heart, in our worries, in our goals, in the dailiness of life that may be causing us to soar or may momentarily be draining us. In other words, *we need not have any answers* when we sit down to talk with each other. We can just share. We want to inform from our heart.

Imposed quick-fixes are not what we're after here. Sharing what's going on, with the vulnerability of not knowing how to fix it, invites the problem-solving skills of *both* partners into the conversation, and that's what we want.

As noted in the previous chapter, we're not looking to set up a communication habit between us that's really about venting. That doesn't solve anything, and it doesn't get us any closer to intimacy, which, by the way, is what we're creating a foundation for in communication.

We don't want to create a summit-meeting experience in which one person dumps all of his or her angst on the other regularly, or brings up every hurt feeling and disappointment from the past ten years, and then expects the other to just take it because we're supposed to be "communicating." That's not mutual, and it's not fair.

Nor do we want to keep ignoring the elephants in the room, putting our head in the sand and hoping against hope that the impact of worries and concerns will simply dissipate and go away. (They won't, by the way. They'll just deaden our sex life.)

These approaches to challenges will breed distrust and unhappiness, as well as transmit a feeling that somehow our partner is not making us happy. Make no mistake about it, our partner will feel that distrust. Avoidance tends to breed an irrational fear that we have no ability to solve problems, which usually is not true. Brooding about how our marriage can't handle trouble can often be an excuse for not developing the chops to speak up or the ability to set some boundaries in the ways we allow ourself to be spoken to when difficult things do come up. Put more simply, we're afraid, so we make excuses instead of finding ways to speak up.

To counteract these going-awry "talking" experiences (and we have all had them), we have to find a healthy mechanism for speaking out, for sharing what's going on within our own heart in a constructive way. That means we need a strong, yet flexible, structure that will allow us each equal time to talk, to listen, and then to discuss what we've shared—a way to comment on or accommodate thoughts, problems, or concerns.

Taking action means we're listening

Going back to our discussion about giving, communicating with our partner is going to require something of us. It's going to ask that we not only listen and nod, but that we take some actual action in the world to shore up our relationship in the places where it's sagging, noting we *each* will have areas to work on. We're not talking about having one partner complain about the other, and then expect, because there was some "sharing," that the other partner should immediately hop to it and comply with all requests. That's not a mutual setup, and it's not realistic.

My husband used to be painfully shy, and he was an avoider where problems were concerned, particularly in our marriage. He would keep things in for months, sometimes for years, and then suddenly something would burst of his mouth that he was angry or concerned about, and he expected me to immediately do whatever he wanted because he finally opened his mouth and spoke up. No discussion, no agreement creation. There was no mutuality in it; no "we" in the process. It drove me nuts.

On the other hand, I would come to him with the attitude of a therapist—an unemotional, here's-the-problem-and-here's-what-we-must-do-to-solve-it lobbyist. I offered no vulnerability, none of my true fears or concerns, so my husband didn't get to know me any better as result of my attempts to communicate. That didn't work either.

Since neither of us liked to be told what to do, these approaches landed us face-first in the mud every time.

Instead, what we want is a setup that allows us to have a calm, open, adult conversation about how we're each doing in our marriage and in our own life. We want to clue our partner in on what's happening in our heart—the real stuff that's wandering around in there from day to day, governing our words and our actions. We can't get to this in the rushed, brusque, information-giving conversations we have in our busy life. We want to deepen our experience together, not distance ourselves from each other.

We need a simple way to do just that: to speak up, to listen—each in turn—and to problem-solve and accommodate for our marriage's sake.

Be willing to talk—and talk nicely

One day I was talking to a friend, a software engineer, about a big glitch in our state's health insurance delivery system. He said that if there is no "hotshot crew"—a group who listens to customer's experiences and follows those experiences through until they find the glitches and fix them—then the whole system stays broken. That's true of marriage, too. Though we don't want to think of our communication time together as always having to be about fixing things—it can just as often be about sharing our gratefulness about how lovely things are—we do need a structure for talking regularly that allows us to communicate about what's really going on, whether it's challenging or grace-filled.

But first we need to set a few ground rules for talking. Communicating needs to be a productive experience. We're not setting up a system to talk to each other as if it's a boxing ring.

If you need to vent, your marriage is *not* the place to do it. If that's your deal—you've got a head of steam on every problem or concern that comes up—then you need a therapist, a wise friend who'll listen as you take a weekly walk, a support group, or a clergy member who can hear you and provide some guidance to help you manage your stress responses.

I am not encouraging you to approach your partner with the idea of regular communication so you can dump your stress and angst upon him or her. What we're after is deeper intimacy—greater communication that leads to deeper caring, which, in turn, enhances our commitment and our closeness. So before we talk about how to set up a regular communication time, we need to agree that the back-and-forth we're talking about here is to *help encourage intimacy.* Meaning, it needs to be respectful, mutual, kind, and open-hearted.

Genuine communication consists of listening, sharing, and accommodating. It is an equal and free-flowing movement between two partners of deepening understanding, and we want to keep that guideline in mind when we sit down with each other and talk.

Galvin and JaeLin

JaeLin and Galvin's major challenge was obvious in our first coaching session. JaeLin is a very quiet spirit and tended to barely speak up about her concerns or emotions, while Galvin demonstratively and exuberantly shared his feelings, pressing for responses from his wife.

When JaeLin refused to respond to Galvin's pressing, he became more and more frustrated, a pattern they both admitted had been creating standoffs between them.

They knew they were in trouble—they had been particularly angry with each other in the past few months—and they wanted to work through their standoff positions, particularly since it was shutting them down sexually. They hadn't had sex for three months, and they both were dissatisfied with being distanced from each other intimately and in their daily communications.

In a session with their therapist, they were asked to address their different communication styles, and although they now had a better understanding of how they were different in their cultural heritage and communication expectations, they still didn't feel like they had enough *strategies* to solve the problem in the

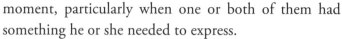

moment, particularly when one or both of them had something he or she needed to express.

JaeLin felt bowled over with Galvin's quick and emotional responses whenever she tried to get words out of her mouth, and Galvin felt like he was "alone on an island, yelling across the water to get my wife to just talk to me."

They agreed that they wanted to learn some simple, no-digging-up-the-past, in-the-moment strategies that could help them communicate and be close. Since sex had shut down between them as a result of their communication breakdowns, we needed to address their communication before anything else. They needed to clear the air so intimacy was possible.

We worked on mastering the Couch Talk style of communicating (as detailed in this chapter).

The deal JaeLin and Galvin made in order to begin was straightforward: they would not talk about intense feelings, issues, or big decisions unless they were having a Couch Talk, and they would only have one per week for thirty minutes. Galvin jumped in and said, "You expect me to get everything I need to say out of me in ten minutes a week?" At which JaeLin visibly crumpled in her chair, and said to me, "See?"

I shared my own marital experience, which is that I needed to realize that for the quieter partner in a marriage—which in mine is my husband—long, involved discussions about feelings more often than not shut him

down. In our first marriage, they often led to a one-sided barrage of me talking *at him* the more upset I got. No listening, no pausing.

For the more verbal partner in a marriage, the quieter partner's reticence can become an opportunity to fill the space with more and more talk, running right over the need to listen or adapt to our spouse's needs.

For JaeLin and Galvin, who were suffering with that dynamic, some equal, but limited, sharing time was in order.

After four weeks of Couch Talks, I met with JaeLin and Galvin again. JaeLin reported that it was hard at first to trust that Galvin wouldn't interrupt her during her ten minutes of sharing with him, but after the first two tries she began to relax. "He started out barely able to keep quiet," she told me, "so it was hard for me to watch that and try to talk. I had to look down sometimes or look away."

I had given Galvin the instruction to *not interrupt*—not with words or even sighing, noises, or big facial responses—to think of the process as a chance for JaeLin to just let her feelings float into the air for a while before he formed or expressed his response. The object, for both of them, was to listen and think about what the other was expressing. To *consider* what was being said.

Galvin said, "This Couch Talk thing made me realize how much I interrupt her. I just can't keep my mouth shut! I always thought it was her upbringing—you

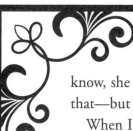
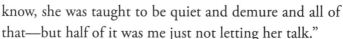

know, she was taught to be quiet and demure and all of that—but half of it was me just not letting her talk."

When I asked how the ten-minute discussion time at the end of the Couch Talk was going, JaeLin said, "It's better. I think the fact that he's listening to me in my ten minutes has helped us both realize that we have to participate half and half. I'm speaking up more, and he's listening more. It's definitely better."

After two months, I gave them another assignment: if they had a big decision to make, they could add a Couch Talk specifically for that issue, for no more than thirty minutes at a time, at the request of either partner. The one caveat, agreed to by both, was that if Galvin needed to process issues emotionally, he'd do so first with a clergy member, therapist, friend, or in a support group so he didn't ramble or steamroll over JaeLin in their Couch Talks.

Now that they were communicating better and listening to each other, they wanted to have sex again and began trying the Naked Date.

JaeLin said, "I guess I never realized that me not speaking up was hurting him. I felt overwhelmed when we tried to talk, so I shut down. Talking this way opened us up. I feel like we can breathe together again."

"I'm just grateful," Galvin said, "because I was doing this to other people—not just my wife. This whole equal-sharing thing has made me wake up, and, for sure, it's already made our marriage so much better."

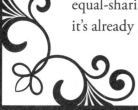

Give up your ships-passing-in-the-night approach to communicating

Everything in marriage conspires to rob us of our ability to spontaneously create intimacy. Our jobs, our kids, our obligations, our duties, our homes, our need to take care of our bodies—all of these are pressing for our time, our mental bandwidth, and our ability to juggle the pieces of our busy lives.

The same is true for communication. If we're ever going to get to a place where we're truly sharing and listening in our marriage, we have to give up our ships-passing-in-the-night approach to talking to each other.

We all know what I'm talking about here. His head is deep in emails as his spouse is trying to get his attention to find out where to pick up the kids. She's chopping tomatoes and pulling a casserole out of the oven as her partner is recounting the stuff he needs from her for the upcoming meeting with the tax accountant. She's running out the door for her evening class while he's asking when they can go visit his father who just got out of the hospital. It's a barely attentive communication style we've adapted in our busy lives—it's filled with logistics and dates and the daily sharing of duties, obligations, and information that neither of us is really paying close attention to.

That means personal, intimate communication is not going to happen unless we set it up. Just like our intimacy, if we don't plan for it, we're not going to get it. Unless we're willing to set some regular time aside to listen and talk to each other, we will never find the agreement and understanding that we're looking for—the kind that leads to a happy intimate life.

Marriage—the way it's constructed in our current timeline—is never going to offer us the free-flowing, unbounded, spontaneous time to communicate with each other one-on-one unless we arrange it and take it. Here's a suggestion for how to do it.

Set up a "Couch Talk"

We talked about setting aside a regular weekly time for intimacy, romance, and sex, and being willing to work on offering more affection to our partner. Now we're going to add a half hour to our schedule to communicate. It's called a "Couch Talk."

A Couch Talk is exactly what it sounds like: it's a half hour set aside each week for the two of us to sit down face-to-face and talk. That's it. The only requirement: turn off all the phones, make sure the screens of all electronic devices are off, step aside from our responsibilities to kids and parents and jobs, and then take thirty minutes to *connect and communicate.*

When I first requested a Couch Talk from my husband, he balked—loudly. We already had a Naked Date, some sex play, some set-aside time for romance, and we were working on more attentive affection. Now I wanted to sit down and *talk?* "Yes I do," I said, "because here's what happens to me when we don't sit and face each other: I have stuff going on in my life and heart that I haven't shared with you, and it ends up coming out of my mouth sideways in short quips—often with more sharpness than I intend. I won't tell you the truth of what's really going on with me unless we're sitting still, looking at each other, because I can't find it in my heart when we're on the run."

That resonated with him. I also knew that since he's a quiet person, he wouldn't come forward with a lot of his feelings unless we set aside some time to think about them and express them in a still moment.

Lastly, I knew we needed a mechanism for talking about things when something came up that was troubling to either one of us, to be able to say, "Hey, hon. Can we have a Couch Talk this morning?" That tool offered us a way to talk calmly and be heard. It's a way to find each other, to create some intimacy and agreement when things come up.

Let's say you agree in theory that the Couch Talk is a good idea for regular communication. How do you set it up? How do you make it work for your marriage?

Just like the Naked Date, the Couch Talk benefits from a regular, weekly time. That said, we're not looking for this to consume whole hours. That was my husband's rule: he was willing to keep our agreement to talk and check in with each other each week, *but only for a half hour.* That guideline kept our talks from turning into summits and allowed us to move into our day and find some fun and relaxation on our Sunday mornings—the time we chose.

To honor that time limit, we do three things:

1. We choose a day and a time.
2. We use a timer.
3. We take turns speaking—ten minutes for me, ten minutes for him, and ten minutes for discussion. Each week we alternate who goes first.

The setup is that simple: thirty minutes every week, by the timer, divided into ten-minute increments. If the timer goes off in the middle of something, we wrap up in a few short seconds or table the discussion until the following week. We don't stress out if we miss a week—we just reschedule a time during the week, or if everything goes to hell, we pick it up the following week.

You may be thinking, *Yikes, there's no way I'm going to get out everything I want to say to my spouse in ten minutes.* But the truth is, we don't want you to. If you haven't been speaking up or truly communicating with your spouse, I guarantee you that he or she will not be able to digest everything you've been holding onto in one gargantuan talking session. The ten-minute guideline gives each partner the dignity to have a good long week to process what's been shared.

We don't want to blast our partner—essentially flattening him or her with everything we've been upset about so that he or she never wants to have another talk again. Again, here we want to apply the Love Sandwich: saying something we appreciate, then something we have concerns about, then finishing with something appreciative. The ten-minute guideline helps us do that.

The good news is, with a ten-minute timeline governed by a timer, we will get good at thinking and expressing our concerns and thoughts in ten-minute increments. That skill—brevity, directness, couched by kindness—will serve us in every realm of communicating in our lives. It's a brilliant little strategy that helps train us to get to the heart of things quickly, simply, and calmly.

The more we do the Couch Talk, the more we feel the benefits of it. We get closer, more trusting, better able to weather everything from problems to heightened joy. Our capacity as a couple grows, and that draws us nearer to each other. We feel that we have each other's back, not just physically or financially, but *spiritually*. That, all by itself, will help to build a healthy sex life.

That's the essence of a Couch Talk: easy, face-to-face, disconnected-from-obligations communication in which we can bare our hearts a bit and let each other in on how we're doing. It's a shortcut that gets us in to the communication we need to have without a lot of muss and fuss: short and sweet, but full of the truth of what's going on inside us.

Guidelines and good news

The object of the Couch Talk is not to solve all of our marriage's troubles in one thirty-minute sharing. Though some problem-solving will get done, the goal here is much broader. The Couch Talk is an opportunity to let our partner in on how we're doing, what we're struggling with, and what accomplishments or pleasures we've been moving through during our week. It's an intimacy tool that helps us create closeness and lets each of us have the floor for a bit to talk about what's moving us or challenging us.

When we do that—when we sit down with a quiet spirit and share with each other—it tends to breed understanding and compassion between our own heart and our partner's. It tends to clue us in on why he or she is behaving in particular ways, and it helps us offer support where we can to lighten our partner's load. It also lets us off the hook a bit, giving us some breathing room for our normal human emotion in relation to our own life experiences. It helps us let our guard down, so we stop trying to be perfect and put-together all the time. When we're being honest and humble like that, it helps to bring us closer.

There's another part of the Couch Talk that helps to fuel closeness between partners: it's a wonderful tool for sharing appreciation with our partner.

When my husband and I first began our talks, we were just getting back together after a divorce and a long separation and there were lots of misunderstandings that needed to get cleared up each week until we found our way. Later, though, there were often Sunday mornings when we had no real issues to discuss, so instead we spent our time expressing how blessed and happy we felt by the gifts of our marriage and each other's actions. This is a beautiful way to use the Couch Talk, too. It doesn't have to be about problems or issues.

However, some personal or existential challenge or some marital or familial need, goal, or problem will usually show up, because that's just how life is. We're always being asked to grow and learn, expand and overcome. We want to be able to share where we are with all of that, giving our spouse a clue to what we're going through, so our normal human challenges don't end up blocking our intimate life.

Choose a time to implement your own Couch Talk. Start simply and with modest expectations. Be respectful and open, and be appreciative of your partner, even when there are issues to bring up. Set a day and a time, use the timer, speak for ten minutes each, and then discuss a bit. Keep the focus on present-moment feelings—how you're each doing *this week* in your marriage and in life—then, watch how your love life blossoms.

More about the Love Sandwich

If one partner is always gobbling up all the air in the room with trouble, never offering any room for joy, gratefulness, or ease, then the other will be less likely to want to return to talking. Marriage is a delicate balance, and we need to treat it gently and lovingly.

Using the Love Sandwich means we say something nice and appreciative about our marriage or the situation we're communicating about first, then we speak our business, and then we wrap up with something kind. We literally sandwich our concerns in between our appreciation. While this might feel as if we're playing a game, or trying to work the room, it actually speaks to a basic human emotional response: we respond better to requests when we know we're appreciated and loved. It's just the way we're wired.

The Love Sandwich is simple imagery to help us remember that when there's trouble, or when we have a request, we'll gain much more ground with our partner by sandwiching it in between our honest love and appreciation.

Sometimes communicating is like open-heart surgery

One of the things I was truly terrible at in my first marriage to my husband was weathering trouble. Whether it was bringing it up, talking about it, or finding strategies for it, I was awful at it. I didn't understand the nature of problem-solving with my husband and I often stunted the conversation with my know-it-all nature, sending our trouble back to its buried, ignored, and marginalized state.

Here's how that played out. My husband and I both knew that we loved each other, and we wanted to be different from other couples who argued and fought, so we avoided the tough conversations. That is, until they reached a breaking point, and then I would speak up. It drove me crazy that I always had to be the one to speak up, so I came to our conversations with angst and with a counselor approach: Here's what's wrong, and here's what we need to do about it right now.

I made pronouncements, offering no room for discussion. In fairness, my husband helped promote this skewed approach by never addressing issues himself and by never bringing up problems.

But our dysfunction ran deeper. When I'd get into therapist mode and try to impose a solution, he would shut down. He would literally not speak to me or touch me for three or four days. That sent the message that if I wanted him to love me, I'd better not ever bring up that topic again. Our issues would then imbed themselves into our marriage more deeply and would rumble from the ground up. We'd ignore them for three or four months, and then the whole cycle would play itself out again, but with more angst.

Issues with lack of money, how to spend it or not spend it, my awful jobs, running up debt, family choices, how to support ourselves as artists and activists—it all got buried. The elephants in the room began to get bigger and more bloated, and pretty soon they were blocking our path to the bedroom—to sex, romance, closeness, and to any kind of fun with each other.

This marital breakdown arc is not unique. Of the many couples I interviewed while writing this book who have had big communication breakdowns, the same result occurs: the inability to talk freely or build the capacity to weather life's issues leads directly to a shutdown in intimacy, specifically in sex.

We need, then, a framework to help us talk through things that will give us a little opening in our hearts and will help us build the capacity to talk things through and also weather the needed changes together. To open up and look at what's going on, ruminate on it, and then see—together—what the next helpful steps might be.

I call that process "Open-Heart Surgery Communicating," and it dovetails quite nicely with our Naked Communication approach.

Open-Heart Surgery Communicating means we *bring up issues with vulnerability,* with no solutions offered. We want to lay the issue on the table, open up the ribs, take a look at that open heart, and see what's going on in there—messy, bound-up, hurt, or confused—and we want to just *look* at it. We want to get comfortable with not knowing what the answer is, being able to ruminate on what the right next step might be.

When we have a large problem, such as careening finances, a troubling division of labor in the marriage, a teenager or partner who's addicted to substances, we need to bring our best self to our Open-Heart Surgery Communication. Our best self will not know the answer immediately, but will benefit from the problem-solving of *two* versus one heart, and we need to make room for our ability to work together.

That means when we have our Couch Talks, or any other problem-solving conversations, we need to approach them with the humility of not having the answers. We can start by saying, "Hon, I know this is a huge problem, and I'm willing to face it, but I don't know what the solution is. Can we think on this long and hard and come back to each other with suggestions?" Then, over the weeks, we do that. We suggest, we turn these rocks over in our hands, looking at all sides of them, seeing how we might smooth the edges so they move downstream and fall away.

If one partner is bringing up the issues more than another in your talks, but you're dealing with them by admitting that you don't know the answers, by making humble suggestions, and by problem-solving with calmness, then don't sweat over who brings it up. Just know that there is progress in humbly addressing things together with serenity and with an adult ethic. We want to be open to solving things together, and we can't do that if we're pushing for a quick-fix or catastrophizing. Humble, open, willing, and with no immediate answers—that's how we want to approach the problems of our marriage.

Show your heart

If we're too afraid to look into our own heart, and we expect our partner to go rumbling around in there when we're not willing to, then we're in real trouble. It's not our partner's job to forage in our spiritual heart for the truth; it's our job. To be brave enough to show our heart is at the very center of a bright and loving love affair.

That's the big news about marriage: it's not some idea or role or image of what we're supposed to be as wives and husbands that's going to save us. It's the baring of our honest, mixed up, frail, quirky, and very human heart that's going to help us build a strong road in the middle with our partner.

That's what marriage is—there's you, there's me, and there's this road in the middle that we build. There really are no set-in-stone guideposts to figuring out how to manage that except listening and paying attention to who we are, to who our spouse is, to how we're each uniquely wired, and to what we can build together.

All of the avoiding, smoothing over, and trying-to-look-good moves we perpetuate with each other are about the outer shell of marriage. It's a pretend life, trying to keep up with the Joneses, and it doesn't work to promote fulfilment. When we play out our marriage to *look good,* without the vulnerable commitment of telling real truths and letting them sit there, big and messy on the table, what we get is *looking good.* We don't get happiness or peace. We don't get the intimacy of a genuine love affair.

Baring our hearts, slowly and deliberately, is how we begin to create the simple ease that communication brings, along with the genuine intimacy it leads to.

What to do if your partner won't speak up

If your partner has a quiet spirit or is a closed-off-from-feelings person, don't bully or push him or her into speaking in your Couch Talks. On the flip-side, don't take up all of his or her speaking time when you're attempting to communicate as a couple. Remember that sharing is a mutual act, and if it hasn't been mutual in your marriage, you'll need time to train each other into an equal ability to open up.

So, what can you do if your spouse agrees to have a Couch Talk but won't share with you?

First, you'll need to allow a period of time for trust to build. Often in relationships in which one person is closed off from feelings, there has never been a safe space to share them instituted long enough for the quiet soul to speak out. That's true both in the marriage and sometimes in the partner's childhood family situation.

I'm not speaking of partners who have been bullied into quietude by controlling partners who verbally and behaviorally don't allow the other partner to have input. For the purpose of this section, I'm going to define the "quieter person" as someone who, for reasons of natal family, nature, or tendency, is naturally more interior. This also applies to people who may be, at first glance, extroverted, but who have had family lives in which their needs were marginalized by needy, difficult, angry, or addictive parents, or other family dynamics. In other words, some partners may have a hard time getting to their real feelings because they were never trained or allowed to have them or share them.

Many adults in our culture don't even know what they feel and have no access to expressing feelings. Though this book is not about the psychological journey of coming to know our emotional state of mind, being married does encompass the need to know ourself well enough to share how we're doing. Sharing ourself is the only way we're going to create the understanding that leads to intimacy.

If your partner says, "I have nothing to say," a number of times during your Couch Talk, ask simple questions that may prompt him or her, such as, "How are you feeling about your mom's illness?" or "What's going on with that deadline you're working on?" and then shut up. Listen. Prompt a little if you need to, but then sit back and wait. Once there's a real space to speak up—a space you're not bolting into whenever there's a pause—your partner will find his or her voice and begin to speak up.

Lorin and James

James and Lorin, by all counts, have the epitome of the American dream. They both have high-paying, achievement-oriented jobs; both are attractive; and two years ago they adopted a three-year-old girl. They're both easy to talk to, funny and witty, and tend toward happy dispositions.

Yet, in their marriage, their communication had broken down, and resentment had begun to build between the two of them, dinging their ability to be close, both intimately and in daily family activities.

James said, "We've always been two driven guys, wrapped up in our careers, making money, and succeeding in a big city, but now, with our daughter, we're a family, and we've got to get our heads out of our behinds if we want this thing to hold together."

When we met, Lorin said they had been "barely grunting at each other" for weeks, huffing and puffing when they passed each other in the house. When I asked if there had been a "what happened," they both admitted to a nasty fight that blew up over Lorin having his head in his phone screen at home.

One night their five-year-old commented on it while she was on the floor putting together a puzzle with James. "Daddy! Put the phone down and play with us!" she said to Lorin, reaching for his device.

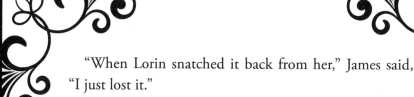

"When Lorin snatched it back from her," James said, "I just lost it."

That simple interchange caused a blaring fight, with both of them "standing in the garage yelling at each other loud enough to rattle the rafters," Lorin recalled.

James said, "I couldn't handle it one more day. When our five-year-old is commenting on it, it's time to do something!"

As two men in a marriage, with a daughter, there are unique challenges in their situation that require sensitivity, but as James put it, "This is basic American marriage crap. You can't have a love affair with your screen and expect to have one with your spouse, too."

Though James is no stranger to Lorin's world—they both direct big media events for corporate clients—he's ten years older, which makes a difference in how they each feel about their careers and their clients. Also, Lorin's work requires him to leave town for several weeks at a time while he supervises gigs, meaning, there are long, unconnected periods of time in the marriage.

When the three of us sat down together, Lorin said, he "didn't understand what the big deal was; James is pushing me away over something stupid."

James's response: "You're pushing yourself away! You're never just in the room with us! We get two-minute intervals. That's if we're lucky."

I explained that this challenge is not unique to them, or to their marriage. Many couples I speak with have one partner who's joined at the hip with a device, and the other partner feels marginalized. This phenomenon is creating agitation across the board in thousands, if not millions, of marriages.

We set in place several communication strategies that Lorin and James could implement to improve their back-and-forth at home. First, whenever Lorin came home from a gig, no matter how long the trip was, both partners agreed that as soon as their daughter was asleep they would sit down with the timer and have a twenty-minute version of the Couch Talk, where they could each focus on and listen to each other, with no phones in the room.

Then, each week, on Saturday mornings, when they were both in town together, they would have their regular Couch Talk. They'd cue up a movie for their five-year-old and go sit in the living room and talk.

Lorin agreed to stop answering his phone between six-thirty p.m. and six-thirty a.m. James wanted him to power down the thing, but Lorin said he couldn't do that. However, he was able to set the phone to do-not-disturb mode, turn off the ringer, and turn down the volume. Then, he had to promise to not go sneaking off to see if there were any "important" texts. Lastly, he agreed to tell his clients—particularly when he signed new contracts—that he was not available after six-thirty p.m., and he assigned an associate to field last-minute emergency calls.

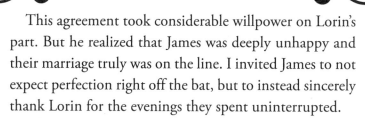

This agreement took considerable willpower on Lorin's part. But he realized that James was deeply unhappy and their marriage truly was on the line. I invited James to not expect perfection right off the bat, but to instead sincerely thank Lorin for the evenings they spent uninterrupted.

After five weeks of practicing the new schedule, an amazing thing happened: all three began having more fun with each other. Lorin said, "I didn't see what I was putting James and our daughter through. But it was like taking a needle out of my arm to stop answering every message. I felt like an addict. I had no idea I was so dialed in to that."

Six months later, they had loosened their agreement to allow Lorin to answer texts in the evenings just before a gig's production delivery date. Since James felt that Lorin had been truly making an effort to be a present participant in their family life, he was willing to make this concession, and the agreement worked.

Lorin said he felt "far better than I used to." He began bike riding with their daughter around the park before dinner, his blood pressure went down by fifteen points, and he dropped eight pounds.

Most importantly, the couples' intimacy was restored, and the humor, wit, and ease came back into their daily family life. James said, "These little agreements saved our asses. We're talking and actually focusing on each other and our daughter now, and I feel like I have my husband back."

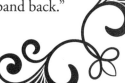

Real worries in the real world

Worries, when they come up, are real for us. They scare us and work on our heart in ways that take our contentment down with them.

By suggesting we use the equal-time approach of a Couch Talk in our marriage, I'm not assuming that real worries will come up equally for each partner. I'm also not saying that one partner may not feel those pressures more than the other, or may not need to express them with more urgency. Things land differently on each of us.

Our Bay Area neighborhood has been going through crazy rent increases, and many people who live near us, and whose incomes are nowhere near high enough to buy a home in this outrageous market, are being forced out of their apartments by their landlord's opportunistic rent increases. People are not only being pushed out of our city, they are being priced out of the whole geographic region. And it's not a false fear—it's really happening to thousands of people.

So my husband and I had a long conversation about how the fear of losing our beloved home is affecting our equilibrium as a couple: we are fielding escalating increases in rent and health insurance each year, while our income is not increasing at anywhere near the same rate, and it's making us more fearful for our future each day.

I have found myself angry and agitated about it, while my husband tends to get silent over it. In our dynamic he trusts more, playing out the good of each day, and I tend to be concerned over the future. And this dynamic can make me crazy. I think, *He doesn't even care. He's got his head in the sand and we're going to get screwed financially and have no place to go.* Because I feel powerless as well as tied geographically to our families, the pressure comes out of me in sideways comments—quiet panic and let's-get-out-of-here desperation that leads me to say things I don't really mean that upset my husband.

When we get to that place, I know the only thing to do is to sit down and talk about the issues, about what we might be able to do to ease the pressure, and hopefully create some options.

I know that sounds pat—we just have to sit down and talk—and I'm well aware that it's often not as easy as it sounds. But since we have a practiced way of communicating now, we can sit down for a half hour with a piece of paper and a pen and sketch out what our options might be if we get priced out of our apartment.

Without having to get overly dramatic and panicky about my fears, we were able to address a short-term, interim set of strategies, and create an emergency plan in case we have to get out fast, as well as develop a few longer-term thoughts about how long we can weather this before we have to jump. In other words, we came up with a *plan* as a couple regarding our housing, and that calmed both of us down. I put the list on our refrigerator so we could peruse it over the next few weeks and keep considering, and we were able to move on with our week without panic.

That doesn't mean we won't wake up in the middle of the night worried, or that we won't be in a flurry of emotion and loss if we lose our home. We will. But being able to get it out of our heads and hearts and discuss some options together assured us that we could weather what comes—unpleasant as it might be. That made us both relax a bit.

Naked Communication doesn't mean everything is solved instantly. It just means we create a path together and a bit of agreement that helps us function and lets us focus on our *loving* while we're fielding the problem.

The next day, we were able to come to our Naked Date with no avoidance and no buried panic blocking our path to each other, and our intimacy helped us feel better about being able to address what's coming next.

That's how this works. We don't have to have the answers. All we need is the confidence that we will find a way, and that's what our Couch Talk and our Naked Communication strategies give us. We're on each other's side, and we're making things right for ourselves and our marriage as best we can.

Present-moment-time communicating

In my own life, in my coaching, and in my books, I always focus on encouragements and strategies that are start-from-today, present-moment tools. No digging up the past. No going backwards. No beating ourself up for what we've done wrong and can't fix. Just begin today to create a new history with better tools and more willingness. And that's also true for our marital communication.

Why do we care if we keep our communication focused on the present moment versus digging up stuff that happened in the past? Because going on an archeological dig of our marriage's failures and letdowns will not help us *now* to become willing to implement the kinds of strategies we're talking about in this book. Meaning, the tools offered here work in short and sweet time frames because we're not bringing the whole trainload of our failures to bear on the current moment.

Now, we could say that's just barreling over a lot of stuff that's deep-seated and festering. But, again, this is not a therapy book for couples who are in serious breakdown. This is a book for couples who know they love each other, but who need some shortcuts to get to the things that promote intimacy in their busy lives, including communication.

We want to have a focus for our communication that supports that idea. And the way to do that is to *just have clarity for today.*

What does that mean, exactly? It means we deal with the challenges at hand, and we don't go back in time and try to settle the score from months or years past.

Did he do something that tanked your finances and you're terribly pissed off about it and can't let it go? Then tell yourself to *start from today* and use the Naked Communication strategies to see what you can come up with to make things better. If you need an apology, calmly ask for one, accept it when it's given, and then move on with what you can both *do.*

Did she have an emotional intrigue with someone at work five years ago, but then she gave it up yet you still can't? Then tell yourself to *start from today* and ask which Naked Marriage principles you can apply so your love and devotion will deepen *now*. That's the idea: communication that leads to action and change.

Start from today is an incredibly hard adage to live by in marriage, particularly when we've been together for a longer period of time. It's even harder to stand by it when we're first beginning our Couch Talks, or when we're in the middle of a fight.

Know that it's difficult, but try to keep a present-moment focus as your goal. We'll delve into this concept in detail in the Naked Money chapter, but I'm encouraging you to keep it in your thoughts as we continue talking about our strategies for communicating.

We want to keep the focus on here and now, so the speaking up, listening, and acting will help us *progress versus regress*.

Fight fairly

The concept of fighting fairly came up in many of the marriage books I researched. It's an important topic, so we're going to address it as simply as we can here.

As we get better at Couch Talks and requests for communication, affection, romance, and regular sex and intimacy, our need to fight regularly often dwindles away. But we're human, and once in a while our irritation is going to bite us in the behind, and we're going to raise our voice, and then, *baboom!* A fight will begin.

Fighting is a mechanism that will get stuff out in the open that's been bottled up, and as such it can be useful. But it can be incredibly hurtful, and when engaged in often, it doesn't promote regular or close intimacy.

Yeah, yeah, I know—there's make-up sex, and that's often grand. But if we're going through cycles of blowing up at each other in order to get things out in the open, we're going to do much more damage than occasional make-up sex can repair. More often than not, after a fight we will end up avoiding each other, brooding, and staying far,

far away from the arms that threw the sharp spears that wounded our heart. Usually, after a fight, we can't find our way back to each other easily for a good long time.

The nasty, harmful things that have been hurled in a fight will fester, and they will block our path to getting vulnerable and naked with each other for sure.

But fights will happen. It's the nature of being with another human being. We want to mitigate how often they happen by having regular Couch Talks and communication sessions, by diminishing the number of eruptions in our marriage so there's an ease that leads us back to a relaxed sensuality.

Here's something I learned over the years in my own marriage: when something's bothering me, it's best to ask my husband for a thirty-minute Couch Talk *sooner rather than later*. Even if I feel foolish—if the issue hasn't really shown itself in its full form, but I'm sensing the arc of it and am worried—I find that speaking up sooner helps prevent fights later on.

In our marriage, we hate to fight. We're both sensitive creatures, and it leaves us both too bruised to function well. We've noticed that it takes us a long time to recover—it dings our ability to do our work, it robs us of focus on our tasks in the world, and takes away our ability to care for ourselves and each other—so we do all that we can to clear things up before they get to a breaking point.

But when we do fight, we have learned to fight fairly.

Fighting fairly encompasses three straightforward things:

1. Keeping the topic matter to the issue at hand.
2. Listening as well as talking, even when voices are raised.
3. Observing a strict rule of no name-calling, no below-the-belt comments or bullying.

Keeping the topic matter to the fight at hand means we don't drag up every hurt or slight our partner has ever committed and say, "Well, *you* did this, so why should I listen to you tell me what *I* did that hurt you?!"

Stop trying to build an army on your side of the fence ("My mother says you're just wasting our money and you don't have a clue how to manage it!") or make accusations that categorize your partner ("Why is it my fault? All you and your friends do is go to exercise classes and shop! You never contribute a damned thing to this family!")

Instead, try to find the heart of the topic, and if you're going to fight, fight from that place. In the context of fighting fairly, that means we say things like, "I'm losing it because we never have any money and we're always in debt! I feel like I'm trapped!" and, then a response of, "Then why are we always buying things that we can't afford? I can't stand it, and I don't want to do it anymore!" That's topical fighting. It's *on-topic*, and it's outing something that needs to get outed.

Listening as well as talking, even in a fight, means we don't bully our partner by rapid-fire bulldozing as we speak, even at higher decibel ranges. We take a breath. We get out a sentence, and then we *listen*. Sure, listening while we're fighting is hard to do.

But here's the kicker, the importance of what we're after in fair fighting: *try to listen for the heart of your partner's message, not the way he or she is saying it.* Don't take issue with the way your partner says something as a way to avoid the heart of it. For example, when your partner says, "I'm losing it because we never have any money and I feel trapped!" don't say, "Oh, we *never* have any money? What was that car last year? What was our kids' camp tuition and our vacation last summer?" Or, worse, "So now I'm *trapping* you? Now I'm your *jailer* in this marriage?!" Avoid that nonsense. Listen for the *feeling*, the real upset, the stuff that needs to be addressed.

I cannot say this strongly enough, whether in fighting or communicating, *hear* what your partner is saying, even if he or she is not expressing it perfectly, or even very well. *Do not* take issue with the way he or she says it. Hear the core of it, or you will block your partner's willingness to ever talk to you again. Your marriage will fail if you purposely try to stamp out your partner's efforts to communicate with you by derailing the message with eruptions about how he or she worded things, especially in a fight. That strategy is an avoidance tactic used to smokescreen the issues so you don't have to address them. Don't do that! We want to get to the heart of what's not working. That's the object of a fair fight.

There's something else about fighting. Don't think that because the two of you are fighting regularly and *you* think you're "doing fine with it" that your partner is too. If you're the one who tends to lose it, blow up, or bulldoze over your partner's attempts to get something out of his or her mouth, you're going to shut your partner down.

Look into your spouse's eyes while you're yelling and you'll know: you will almost never see joy or ease in your partner's eyes when you're bellowing at him or her. We're all children at heart when we're screamed at: it never works to motivate us, it just hurts. So give it up as much as you can in favor of communicating—each week, in your Couch Talk, applying the "sooner-rather-than-later" approach to problems—and when the occasional fight does erupt, fight fairly.

No name-calling

Lastly—and I really shouldn't even need to say this to couples who know they love each other—no name-calling during fights or at any other time. It wounds. Be an adult, think about what you need to get out of your mouth and heart, and, even when you're upset, don't resort to name-calling.

Name-calling is not cute, it's not kind, and it's not helpful. It's *not* okay. It will not, under any circumstances, help you get back in bed together or create a free-flowing sense of trusting intimacy. And here's the crux of it: who wants to get naked and vulnerable with a person who has decimated our heart, soul, and self-esteem?

Communicating and fighting fairly means we listen, even when temperatures are high and voices are raised. It means we address only the topic at hand, not our whole history. It means we never, ever name-call. Fighting means there's something unaddressed that needs to get addressed, and as adults we behave fairly and we treat it that way.

The request behind the irritation

What we're trying to get good at by using the Naked Communication strategies in this chapter is to speak about things before they blow up and clue our partner in on how we're really doing, and to listen, too. We want to create agreement by looking into our marriage's open and bared heart, even when we don't have any answers.

But irritations will arise, so how can we field them better than we have in the past, before they erupt into fighting? What's the antidote to irritation?

The antidote to irritation is summed up in the simple adage: *What is the request behind the irritation?*

When we have an irritation, we need a framework for speaking up. So ask yourself, before you speak, *What is the request behind the irritation? What, specifically, do I need from my spouse right now?*

That means we stop trying to get the other person to do what we want him or her to do by shaming and blaming, by snipping and snapping, or by avoiding and being passive-aggressive. We instead think through—and *feel* into—what might be causing our upset and what might help, and then we ask our partner for it from that place.

If, for instance, I'm upset because my husband is seemingly unconcerned about our rent and health insurance increases and our inability to pay them with our current income, then I need to speak up about it. But that guideline of speaking up could easily deteriorate into a one-sided blasting that eviscerates him, so I also have to practice some discernment while speaking up. With all of the fear and worry I feel about this issue in my throat, I could easily end up saying, "What's wrong with you? I'm up all night worrying about this, and you fall asleep at the drop of hat like it doesn't matter at all to you! You don't even care that I was up last night crying about this! You don't care about me!!"

Sure, we could say that's a form of speaking up, but it's not going to get me any closer to what I really want: a feeling that we're in this together and that we have some plan for our marriage if we lose our housing.

It wouldn't get me any further if I approached him by saying, "You just have your head in the sand! You *refuse* to deal with this with me! You're going to ruin us!" Now he has to either defend himself, bully back, or shut me out. And nothing gets solved.

In this example, I have to figure out what it is I really need, and then ask for it. Do I want my partner to solve the whole thing for me in one fell swoop? Sure, that would be grand, but he's not in charge of the universe, so I need a more practical request. Do I want him to stay up with me all night worrying? Not really, no. That won't help. What I want is to feel easier about this. What I want is to have a "we" plan, in case we need to move in a hurry. So that's what I ask for: "Babe. Can we have a Couch Talk today and strategize together about what we might do if we lose our apartment? I'm staying up night after night worrying and I need your help."

That's the true request behind the irritation. It's also the communication that will keep us from fighting about something bigger than us that we cannot control, but which we need to have a strategy for in order to feel safe in our daily life.

But just because we make a request of our partner doesn't mean the other person is obligated to say yes. Our partner has the right to say "no." We want to keep that truth close to our heart as we ask for things.

Here's an example. I remember once early in my move to teach yoga instead of working at a higher-paying job, my husband turned to me and said, "It would be nice to have some more money, you know?" I paused, thought about it, and said, "I'd like that too. But I'm never going to be a nonprofit fundraiser again. I just can't do it anymore.

I've accepted that you're not going to suddenly become a banker or a union rep instead of a teacher, and I guess I'd like that same acceptance from you." I said it calmly and kindly, as did he.

He made a request for me to make more money, I heard it as such and said no. I knew that I couldn't do that work anymore and bring happiness and ease to myself or my marriage. I wasn't able to offer him that. But once we discussed it, I *could* offer him the gift of living wholly without debt and money pressure, keeping my promise of living well within our means, and still plan a vacation every year and live happily, appreciative that he was enabling me to live the life I wanted to live.

At the heart of the request-behind-the-irritation idea is kindness. Thinking through what our part is, what we really need in the actual situation or challenge, making it reasonable and adult, and then asking for it calmly and kindly. It's a skill every one of us can work on in marriage, a way of communicating that will help lead us, again and again, back into each other's arms.

CHAPTER SIX
NAKED MONEY

Money trouble kills our sex life

Money issues are at the center of so much trouble in our marriages that we have, as a culture, developed a kind of psychological shorthand for referring to them. We say, rather offhandedly, "He's a train wreck with money," "I'm disastrous with numbers and my husband's just going to have to deal with it," or "We're going to be in debt until the day we die, and that's just the way it is." We ignore, we get brazen and blasé, and many times we're so deadened to the effects money trouble is having on us we barely notice that it's killing our sex life.

We engage in regular, casual side-stepping of our money issues, blaming our partner, dissing our own capabilities, or fatalistically denigrating our marriage with statements like, "We're a disaster financially, but there's nothing we can do about it." Many of us apply a head-in-the-sand approach to dealing with our marital money decisions, and, eventually, that strategy blows up in our faces.

According to the Institute for Divorce (www.institutedfa.com), money trouble is one of the top three causes of divorce in our country. (Infidelity and incompatibility are the other two, and it's telling that money trouble also fuels incompatibility as well.) Look up "causes of divorce" on any Internet search and you'll find money trouble at the top of the list.

So, if we think we can casually sidestep the issues money brings up in our partnership without driving our marriage toward serious divisions or divorce, we are sorely mistaken. Money upsets not only put pressure on us financially, they can also tank our time (because we mistakenly believe that overworking will get us out of our financial hole); our values (because of vague overspending with no clear goals), *and* our intimacy. And if we don't have solid strategies for dealing with them, they can ruin our marriage for good.

But long before we ever get to the brink of a divorce, money trouble will surely kill our sex life. Money issues will drain us, pull us apart, and block us from being close to each other every time. Plain and simple, financial trouble puts so much pressure on us as a couple that we can't find our way back into the realm of each other's arms, let alone get ourselves naked under the bedroom sheets.

Sure, we can sometimes bulldoze over trouble, using sex to blot everything out. But that strategy tends to disintegrate quickly over time and will usually end up leveling our marital landscape.

Trying to be intimate when there's serious financial trouble feels way too vulnerable for most of us. We're angry at our spouse; we're pissed off at our situation; we're touchy and bitchy and furious that we're out of control and can't seem to get a grip financially. That's hardly a mood-setter for allowing our most vulnerable body parts to be touched and stimulated. In fact, many of us who have large, unaddressed money problems will often just go dark on our partner sexually, and we may not even realize that the boxed-up feelings we have concerning our tanking finances are the root of the problem.

We can't ignore these issues and realistically think that we're going to stay close and stay sexual. It's not going to happen with our head in the sand, nor is it going to happen by trying to skate by and shove our money trouble to the side, attempting to breeze by it or even bulldoze over it. Eventually it will trip us up, landing smack-dab in the middle of the entryway to our bedroom, blocking all efforts to get naked and get close.

What we need is a strategy for dealing with money that keeps our communication open, and will help us manage our financial choices simply so they don't take over our life. Particularly if there's debt, financial pressure, or overspending in our marriage, we need a plan that helps create equal participation and responsibility in our decision-making about our money, and is easy to implement.

We need a strategy for *peace* with our finances—a plan, in other words—so that even if everything's not perfectly lined up monetarily, we know what we're doing and can enjoy an open intimate life while we're doing it.

I'm not suggesting that we need to have money perfection before we can generate the financial peace that promotes intimacy. That's not realistic. What we're after is *agreement*—i.e., having a plan that works for us—so we know what we're up to together (and individually) with money, which then allows us to relax and enjoy our married life.

The money-trouble cocktail

If we've been sipping the money-trouble cocktail for a number of years, getting high on spending and then tanking with the bill-paying hangover of that behavior, then the very thought that we could have peace in our money decisions is going to seem like a pipe dream.

I know this very well. My husband and I were there in our first marriage. We broke up largely over our debt, brought about by vague and troubling money choices, and the fallout from that mess. I remember feeling trapped in a corner with my partner over money, but we kept crashing the train by charging romantic dinners on credit cards as a quick-fix, feel-better approach. Later, when the debt-pressure boomerang crashed down on my head and I was still stuck doing jobs I hated, I would go down a dark emotional hole of depression and hopelessness, which dinged not only my mood, but my attitude toward my husband. I was angry, pissed-off, confused, and lost. Not a great cocktail for trying to stay open to my husband intimately.

We each thought the other one wasn't earning enough. Now I know that we never learned to live within our means or learned how to make decisions together where money was concerned. No one had ever taught us these skills. We were floundering, facing drama after drama financially, and it limited our choices, both in life and in our partnership.

In this chapter, we're going to stem the tide of marital disaster that money trouble creates by *creating a plan.*

I'm not saying that we have to have all of our financial ducks lined up perfectly before we can have a good time in bed or some peace in our marriage. Not only is that unrealistic, but it also puts too much pressure on us. But we do need a strategy that brings ease to our money experiences or we will constantly be dinging our intimate life.

We need to learn how to communicate about money within the framework of our marriage.

What we're after is agreement

Here's the most salient point of the approach we're going to take in this chapter: *we're not after perfection; we're after agreement.*

Agreement will calm the waters of our stormy marital money seas. It will ease our hearts, make us respect each other, and allow us to feel responsible to each other. Being responsible doesn't seem like it would be as sexy as saying, "To hell with the bills, let's go to Tahiti on the credit cards!" But, in reality, responsibility works to promote sensual closeness.

How, you ask? Because clarity breeds ease. Having a plan creates mutual respect. It allows us to look over at our partner and feel ease instead of feeling trapped. Easiness is what we need to keep getting close to one another, to keep wanting to get in bed with each other—finding a clear path to each other, each week, unobstructed by trouble.

The sad (and silly) thing about money trouble is it's relatively easy to fix. However, in our imagination, we perceive money issues as a huge boulder that we're barely balancing over our marital heads—a ridiculous, impossible balancing act. It makes us feel trapped, angry, powerless, and helpless. Those feelings *do not,* in any way shape or form, contribute to us getting sexual with each other. In fact, many of the couples I interviewed for this book that had burdensome money, debt, and time issues (e.g., overworking to try to get out from behind the financial eight ball), had not had sex in a year or more.

We don't want, as a coaching client labeled it, "marital bed death." We are entitled to the love we committed to—entitled to the joy and ease that intimacy brings us. If we're in financial trouble, then we've got to help our marriage get these two important things:

1. A plan.
2. A clarity agreement.

Remember, the focus is on *progress, not perfection.* We don't need to have our money perfectly aligned (with a chunk of cash in the bank) before we can have a healthy, vibrant sexual life. What we do need is *agreement,* a strategy, and a simple plan for how to deal with our money.

Own your shared responsibility

The very first thing we need to address when we talk about money issues is our shared responsibility in the mess.

Those of us who have had financial trouble in marriage often tell a story that involves blaming or shaming our partner. It usually goes something like this: "Well, if you just earned more and stopped working that dead-end job then we wouldn't be in this mess!" Or, "It's your fault! If you would just stop all of this goddamned shopping I wouldn't be sweating bullets trying to pay these bills every month!" Or, "Why should I stop spending when you just bought a new motorcycle that we can't even remotely afford?!"

We often engage what I call our "private armies" to shore up our contention that we're right, meaning we bring other people into our arguments to "prove" how righteous we are and that it's not our fault. "My mother told me I should never have married you because you're never going to be a decent provider!" Or, "My friends say you act like an entitled child with money. When are you going to grow up?!"

This doesn't work. It doesn't work to just *think* this stuff either. It's part of the blaming game, and it only gets us stuck deeper in the muck. Rather than being willing to create a strategy to solve the problem, we end up with one foot out the door, blaming our partner for the mess. Intimacy isn't possible while we're in a stand-off with our spouse.

Even if we're completely innocent of overspending or running up debt and we've been sitting silently by, watching our partner break the bank, then guess what? *We are the other half of the problem.* We are the codependent in the mix, sitting by and watching as the train veers off its tracks.

If we've been ignoring the money issues in our marriage, then the onus is on us as much as it is on our partner.

How can we stop playing the blaming game? How can we become willing to look at our money issues dead-on, without any histrionics, blame, or punishing stances?

We have to speak up—without shaming or digging up the past— and talk to our partner about it. Plain and simple.

If money trouble and lack of financial clarity have played a part in troubling your marriage, before you continue reading this chapter, I invite you to make this promise to yourself:

I will be willing to look at what's going on right now with our money, and I won't bring up the past. I will not fight with, shame, or blame my partner over our money trouble. I will take full responsibility for my part in not speaking up, in ignoring and not addressing our issues. I will be willing to start from today and build a new and clear money plan with my partner so our intimacy can flourish.

Give up being right

One of the most powerful things I've ever learned is this: *the need to be right costs me my intimacy with others.*

Think about that for a moment. The mechanisms we use to "prove" that we are right—lobbying for it, convincing, bullying, steamrolling, passive-aggressively controlling—may help us win the immediate battle, but ensure that we will lose the war.

Why? Because when we're hell-bent on being right, we're not listening. As we discussed in the Naked Communication chapter, when we're lobbying like a mad dog for our righteous stances, we're usually trying to shut the other person up (so we don't have to listen to our partner's feelings, needs, and experiences), but also as a way to never have to examine our own behavior. We bellow, get belligerent, or bully, whine, avoid, or control as a means to an end. That end is *the need to be right.*

Be very clear about this point. When we're bringing up money issues with our partner, we're just starting to attempt to create the kind of agreement that will bring peace to our marriage, so we don't want to engage in parental, blame-throwing, controlling, or inventory-taking stances of righteousness. Nor do we want to approach our partner with know-it-all, therapist-like, fix-it-my-way proclamations.

In fact, when we first bring up money issues with our partner, *we should offer no answers at all. Not one.* No thoughts about how you both got into this mess, no finger-pointing about who should be doing what, no "suggestions," which are often just righteous stances clothed as "helpful" thoughts.

We want to give up being right in any way, shape, or form. Instead, we want to approach our partner letting them know how *we* are feeling using a simple "I" statement.

For example, I might say something like, "Hon, I've been so upset about our money trouble for so long, and I'm just bummed out all the time over it. I know there's a big problem here, and though I don't know what to do about it, I want you to know that I'm willing to work with you to find a new way that works for both of us."

Beware of faux I statements that call your partner out, such as, "I feel that you've got your head in the sand about our money issues," or "I know this is a bigger problem for you, but I'm willing to talk about it." We want to say something kinder, more direct, and more honest and clear, with no baiting.

We want to think through how we will first approach our partner and be calm and accepting of *how things are right now,* no matter what the damage level.

Three birds

Let's say we've gotten up the courage and we've thought through our "I feel" money statement to our partner, and we've said it out loud to him or her. What can we expect in terms of how long it will take to sink in? Should we expect our partner to jump right in with complete willingness just because we're now willing?

No. That's not how the human heart works.

Let me share a little story I call "Three Birds to Change a Paradigm" to illustrate the timeline we humans need to accept things we don't want to look at.

Say you're dining at a luxurious home, sitting at a long table, and everyone is elegantly dressed and enjoying a sumptuous dinner. Suddenly, you see a bird fly across the ceiling. You blink, check your wine ingestion, thinking you couldn't have seen a bird, you're in the dining room after all. You think, *Couldn't be,* and you blow it off. Then while chatting with your neighbor at the table, you see it again. *There it is!* You turn to the person next to you and say, "Did you see that? There was a bird flitting across the ceiling!" Your neighbor laughs it off and asks, "How much wine have you had, anyway? There's no bird in here, this is a dining room!" You go back to your conversation and then—*there!*—there it is again! You *know* you saw it this time! "Hey everybody," you say to the diners, "there's a bird in here!"

That's about the speed of emotional recognition you should expect from your partner when bringing up money issues the way we're describing here. You've probably brought up financial trouble before in ways that are less than productive. But this time it's different. This time, *you're calmly stating that you know there's a problem, you know it's a big one, you don't have any answers, and you're willing to find a way together to work on it.*

When you speak like this—from your own willingness and offering a perspective on your feelings—you need to give your partner time for the weight of what you're saying to sink in. You can't expect that he or she will be right on point with you just because you've awakened to the need for change.

Here's the way I use this tool: I speak my truth calmly at least three times over the course of two or three weeks—preferably in three sentences or less—and then I back off, walk away, and let my partner think about it. Then, after the third time, when I can reasonably expect that my partner knows I'm serious about this, and I know I can speak about it calmly, I ask for a Couch Talk so we can begin sharing and strategizing.

As you're beginning to bridge the canyon of your money trouble, understand that you're going to need to speak up, but realize that it will probably take three times before your partner sees the bird.

Just have clarity for today

Once we've set the stage for talking about money trouble, how do we begin? How can we start having a conversation about it with our spouse, particularly if we have been avoiding it for years?

The guideline used in the previous chapter applies here, too: *just have clarity for today.*

This means there is no need to go back in time and clear up who spent how much and when. There is no need to insistently list every money error our partner has ever committed, or conversely to have to field those accusations from our spouse. There is no reason to shame or find fault with our partner in any way. We want, instead, to create agreement *now*, to invent a new sense of peace around our money, beginning from this moment. Going over the past will get us absolutely nowhere.

This is the incredible, magical key to talking about your marital money that will save you from yourself: do not go back and dig up your past spending from the past five years; do not go on an archeological or psychological dig into your childhood or your early adult attitudes about money; do not "process" your feelings about money for your whole adult life and marriage. That nonsense doesn't do anybody any good. The only thing that will change your money life (and your love life) for the better is *action*.

Changed behavior will make us feel better and will open up the landscape of our money choices, and that will put the ease back into our sex life and our marriage. We want to build a new financial history, starting from today, that will support us in every aspect of our choices and our intimacy.

We refrain from delving, from digging, from philosophizing, from psychologizing, from weighing our or our partner's blame in our money distress. *We deal with the exact issues at hand.* No matter what the damage level, we start from today. We commit ourselves to the actions that are going to make a difference, which are going to help us respect each other around our money.

Trust me when I say this: when we start from today, we give our marriage the dignity of a brand-new history—a clean slate, a new start, the beginning of a new kind of agreement that breeds closeness. In a month, two months, three months, we will have a whole new track record and a new platform from which to support our money choices and our family choices. That's powerful.

Esteemable acts of money clarity

When we're willing to have clarity for today, we will, step by step, create a history that's clean, bright, and aired out, and that doesn't come with the weight of every mistake we ever made together. We rebuild, stone by stone, the reverence we once had for each other by engaging in *esteemable acts of money clarity* together, right now.

What in the world are "esteemable acts of money clarity," and how do we get some for our marriage?

First, we use the strategies in this book to calmly talk about our money challenges. We show up without any answers, looking at our financial problems like an open-heart surgery, pulling back the ribs to get a good look at what's going on in there right now. We're going to notice that there's trouble and be committed to changing our approach together. We're not going to dig into the minute details of what's wrong, how it went wrong, or who caused it. We're going to be willing to *not know* how to fix it, and then craft something together that will.

Then, if anything is going to genuinely shift, we've got to get real about the prospect of changing our behavior. What will that look like?

I'm going to give you some guidelines that will help you reach a money agreement. You may choose to not use them, and that's okay, *but you must get a plan of some kind.*

We've all heard the definition of crazy: Doing the same thing over and over again and expecting a different result. So we need to get practical about creating ways to change. We must have a plan—one that's grounded on planet Earth and will actually work in our busy lives and won't suck up tons of time.

There's a statement I use a lot: *Vagueness creates drama; clarity creates peace.* We want peace for our marriage, so we need clarity—practical, implementable, feet-on-the-ground, money clarity in a plan that we can live with.

Alberto and Elise

Alberto and Elise met twelve years ago at a local elementary school where they both work. She's a kindergarten teacher, and he works on the construction and maintenance crew for the school district.

"I remember when I first saw her," Alberto said. "I was up on the roof repairing a leak, and I saw this beautiful redhead walking to the school activity room with a single-file line of five-year-olds behind her, just like ducklings. I was a goner."

Elise remembers the same moment: "I looked up, and there was this dark, Latin guy with strong legs and mussed hair up on the roof, and I thought, '*Who* is that?'"

Two years later, they married and rented a small house in their town. Since they both have modest incomes, they agreed to always pay off their credit cards and never run up balances. That worked for the first couple of years . . . until they had twins.

When they first came to me, their twins were six years old, and the couple had racked up significant debt, taking a big chunk out of their monthly incomes. Though neither liked to fight, they had had a couple of screaming doozies, and that scared them both enough to become willing to change how they were handling their money.

"I don't want to divorce this man over money," Elise said.

"That seems like a total waste," Alberto said. "I know we're not getting along the way we used to, but she's still the only person I want to be with, so we have to *do* something."

Neither one had received any training from family or at school on how to manage money, particularly as a couple living on modest incomes, so as their expenses increased, they had no strategies to deal with the changes.

They admitted that money trouble was taking the joy out of raising their kids, and worse yet, it was making them edgy with each other, "sucking the sexual desire right out of us," Alberto said.

We began right off the bat to craft a spending plan agreement for them based on their circumstances. Though it took several meetings for them to agree to cut up their credit cards and live only on cash, they eventually canceled the accounts. "I'm terrified to do this. I just don't see how in hell we're going to live without the cards. What if there's an emergency?" Elise asked.

I said that the trouble with the "emergency" argument is that it's usually *non-emergency* purchases that end up going on the cards—one spouse figures he or

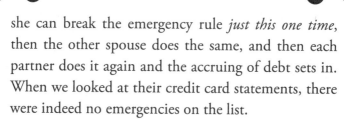

she can break the emergency rule *just this one time,* then the other spouse does the same, and then each partner does it again and the accruing of debt sets in. When we looked at their credit card statements, there were indeed no emergencies on the list.

We did some simple downsizing of expenses and bills, incorporating the suggestions in this chapter, and we came up with a clear and workable daily spending plan that included a bill-paying and savings plan with specific amounts for each partner's daily needs. In the first three months, I suggested they just pay their credit card balance minimums until they got used to living within their cash income. Then, in month three, they were able to adapt a bit to cover eighty dollars more than their minimums, agreeing to not *ever* add anything to the balances.

"This is a big promise," Alberto said, "but I feel like it's the only way we're going to get the happiness we had back. We've got to stop letting money make us crazy."

In the fourth month they had a genuine emergency: Alberto's dental crown cracked in two and their dentist said it was going to cost them seventeen hundred dollars to fix it. A week later, Elise accidentally left the dome light on in her car and blew out the battery, and the shop found that her electrical system needed an additional four hundred dollars' worth of work.

With a little coaching, they agreed to not panic and to get *three comparison quotes* for the services they needed. I suggested they check out the local dental school, which they did, and Alberto was able to get his tooth fixed for five hundred dollars, the exact amount they had in their reserve savings account after three months.

The car was a bigger problem, and since they only had two hundred dollars in their new car repairs savings account they didn't know what to do. Then Elise's brother-in-law proposed a trade: if she and Alberto would take care of their nephew for a week so he and his wife could get away, he'd fix the car for free, including the battery. So that's what they did.

But the larger story is not about the details of their money stuff. The larger win was that the couple was now able to make money decisions together without drama.

"I guess I'm kind of shocked," Elise said, "that after all the anger we've been dumping on each other this past year, we kind of sailed through these things this time. Having some money agreements made it so much easier."

A month later, we talked about what they had learned. When a money problem comes up—and they always will in a marriage—Elise and Alberto now had

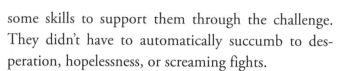

some skills to support them through the challenge. They didn't have to automatically succumb to desperation, hopelessness, or screaming fights.

They now had clarity with the cash they were earning, they knew what expenses they needed to cover and had a plan to fund them, they had some modest savings, and they had a commitment together to keep debt-pressure out of their life. They were also willing to find creative solutions to money issues, even in emergencies. Those simple agreements and strategies made them feel more relaxed with each other, they were fighting less, and, most importantly, their intimacy had been restored.

When I asked what they noticed about the changes in their marriage, Alberto said, "You know, it's not perfect. It's still going to take us at least five years to get out of the debt we ran up, but we're not fighting about it anymore. We're paying it off slowly, and we're not adding to it. In the meantime, we're actually living better, I think, because we're just happier without all that guilt and blame."

Elise said, "That terrible pressure's gone. I feel like I *like* him more now because of the changes we made. And anything that gets me my sex life back has got to be good."

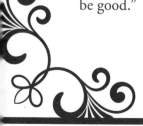

What's a money plan doing in an intimacy book?

I'm a big believer in the practical. My approach is to provide easy shortcuts to apply good ideas in a few-minutes-a-day time frame.

Although it may seem divergent in a book about intimacy to stop and talk about how to craft a money plan, it's actually not, and here's why. If you haven't been able to figure out how to clear up your money issues on your own, what good does it do for me to encourage you to do it without offering a plan to help?

When I was deep in debt, desperately reading personal finance books to try to salvage my finances and my life, many authors said, "Get out of debt; it's a bad idea," yet didn't offer me any tools for getting out. They'd talk about investments or retirement or some other financial topic, as if I could just figure out how to live debt-free on my own.

Instead of leaving you high and dry, I'm going to offer some step-by-step instructions for getting out of the deep, dark forest of debt: the Naked Money strategies that have worked to create peace in my own marriage. My couples' money-agreement plan, which includes a five-minutes-a-day spending plan, is unrivaled at creating money peace between two married people.

In the eleven years that my husband and I have been using this simple approach, *we have never had a fight about money.* In our first marriage, money standoffs led us to divorce. Now we have money decisions, *but we don't have money drama.* We still have financial challenges, but we have peace in our marriage because we have a plan and an agreement, which means money trouble no longer blocks our intimacy or our sex life.

I am living, breathing proof that the strategies I'm about to share with you work. They work to get clarity, to create agreement, and they also help to define division of labor in marriage. By using them we will learn to give up micromanaging each other (a huge plus!) and to fund the things that are meaningful to us as a couple, as well as individually.

The truly brilliant thing is that these strategies work to restore mutual respect, with a bright and lush return to free-flowing intimacy. That's a promise.

When we have a plan for our money, everything settles down. When we settle down, we can get back to what's important. Namely, offering love, desire, and affection to each other.

Time and money: a volatile stew

Before we jump into our couples' money strategies I'd like to say a word about time and money. Money trouble is bound up in the hours we think we need to spend working (working *more*), as well as the stress we feel about running faster, putting in more hours, and trying to dig ourselves out of a money hole. That additional time away from home adds a burden to both our marriage and our family life.

With one or both partners becoming largely more absent as money pressures grow, the marriage doesn't stand a chance. Our stress-cocktail becomes stronger and more intense, and not only do we feel the crush of being pressed to the wall in our family finances, now we're barely ever seeing each other, let alone finding the time to be intimate. So, as we're crafting a clear money plan in this section, it will also help us address our issues with time.

Why are money and time bound up together? Because our perception is that if we could just work a little harder or a little longer, possibly getting a bigger pay raise, then at least *some* of our money issues would fade away. We mistakenly buy into the idea that more hours, and thus more money, might take the financial pressure off our marriage. We work longer, coming home with no energy for our spouse or family, and we say, "It's just these six months, babe," and then we dive back into the work-focused arena with nary a nod to our marital life. Six months turns into a year and a half, which turns into three years, and then six, with no end in sight. By then—particularly if we have debt or a lack of financial clarity—our marriage is on the rocks.

We can default to our old excuses, saying that we have to have a crazy work schedule in order to survive, that that's how life is right now in our timeline, and there's nothing we can do about it but to just keep swimming upstream as hard as we can to keep from being taken down by the financial riptides of modern life. But that's not going to create the intimacy we crave, nor will it promote peace in our family life.

The only thing that's going to create the intimacy and financial peace we crave is to get clarity with our money. So if you're still telling yourself that you can dig yourself out of money trouble by simply earning more or working more hours, you're mistaken. Overspending and "debting" are what's known as "process addictions," meaning, they occur no matter what the level of our earning is. When we have a lack of clarity in our marital money, earning more will almost always mean spending more—and racking up more debt if we're used to using credit cards to live—unless we get a plan that can interrupt the cycle. (I can absolutely attest to this truism from the couples I have coached.)

We do have a workaholic ethic in our American corporate structure, and our bosses and corporate entities have been slow to create structures that allow for the flexible needs of running a family as well as maintaining two jobs. But we buy into the need to overwork so we can earn more. Add overspending, running up debt, and not living within our means to this mix, and it's not only a sex-killer, it's often a volatile time bomb just tick-tick-ticking in the background of our hearts, waiting to explode and destroy our marriage.

Let me be clear. *If we want to have a regular, connected, and close intimate life, then we need to have a plan for our money and our lifestyle choices.*

Am I saying that we have to be completely out of debt and firmly on solid ground financially or have a stress-free timeline before our sex life can flourish? No. What I am saying is that we need a *plan*, an agreement, and a clarity strategy with our money, or we will most surely end up in the kind of financial trouble that takes our sensual life out at the knees.

We want to shift the conversation in our marriage from how much money we have, or how much we think we're supposed to be making, to the *nature of our choices*.

Being clear about our money means we open up the realm of the choices we can make together—that's the focus here. Make no mistake about it, being able to make money, lifestyle, family, time, and even division of labor choices together, with clarity, absolutely has the power to reinvent us sexually and amorously.

"More than enough" can still spell trouble

One last note before we explain the couples' money plan. Some couples don't have to worry about how much money they earn, but most of us do. Even if you're one of those couples who's got plenty of cash, don't think that this challenge of making money choices together doesn't apply to you. It does.

One partner may have earned or inherited plenty of money, so there may be no worries about having enough to live well. But in such marriages, one spouse is often infantilized, taken care of like a child, with no money responsibilities—a don't-worry-your-pretty-little-head approach. That, too, can kill our sex life. Partners need to make choices together monetarily for one simple reason: doing so evens the playing field. If one partner always holds the decision-making power, and one partner is always dependent, it will rob the marriage of an equal interplay of power, which in turn will ding our sex life. The biggest of our marital decisions will involve funding our family life and choosing how to live, and we should each take part in those decisions.

That doesn't mean that each partner has to earn the same amount in order to avoid money trouble, or that both partners have to have jobs. I'm saying that equal, adult *choices* in money and lifestyle decisions breed easy intimacy. It harms us sensually when we're not responsible together; it enhances us sensually when we are.

Why does money work that way on our sex lives? I can offer some theories, but the upshot is clear: money decisions and power go hand in hand in marriage, and when we're able to make choices *together,* what we get is a better sex life. There is a direct relationship between our ability to make decisions as a couple—to find values-agreement and then act on those agreements—and having a rich and vivid intimate experience.

No matter the level of our financial strata, we all need a money plan of some kind if we want to stay close.

Be willing

Willingness is a weird commodity. It doesn't often look like how we think it should. It's not a sweet and rational discussion about "needs" and "wants" and then an, "Okay, hon, that sounds fine" response.

Most often, willingness involves *not knowing*, and then honestly and humbly trying. We have to explore and craft and begin to construct something a little at a time. We need to try things, fail, and then try again to see what really works. We have to invent ourselves, building and hammering things into place and sometimes taking it all apart and starting over.

Willingness for my husband and me meant we had to shut up and really listen when the other person was talking. It meant we wrote notes and pasted them up on mirrors to remind ourselves what the other person needed and wanted. It meant we had to have a strategy for talking each week, a plan for our money, a scheduled time for romance and intimacy. Willingness meant we had to begin to engage in more than generosity. We had to be giving.

We found that for our marriage to work, *really* work, both of us had to be ready to change. Noting our fears of facing our money problems, we still had to ready ourselves, because looking at your money together requires willingness.

I remember my mother and father having an awful money fight that occurred in a persistent pattern. My mother had a chunk of money coming in each month from a trust that amounted to at least one-third of our family's income, and she—believing "this is what women are supposed to do"—turned it over to my father, who handled the finances. As time went on, she began to approach him, asking to sit down and go over the family money choices. He would say, quite belligerently, "You can't understand this stuff!" She would persist, and they would finally sit down. About ten minutes in, when she asked a question, he would bellow, "See! I told you that you can't understand our money! It's my job!" In response, she would cry and run out of the room, because there was absolutely no willingness there. The whole thing would repeat itself three months later.

What I didn't know then is that my father was trying to manage the balls-in-the-air of our family's overspending, as well as a lack of savings for college and other family needs. As far as I can tell, he was trying to block anyone questioning his own unhealthy behavior, as well as covering for the vagueness my mother had with spending money. My mother was a willing participant by not standing up strongly and refusing to go along with the status quo (as hard as that would have been). This dynamic definitely contributed to my parents' divorce.

We cannot be belligerent; we cannot try to hold all the cards so we can control the money landscape; we cannot yell and scream and bully to get our way. We also cannot crumble at the first roadblock; we cannot allow ourself to be run over just because our partner bellows or tries to control. If we do, we will end up completely shut down with each other or in divorce court.

Willingness means we admit our fear and show up humbly anyway, without answers. We get a plan that includes input from *both* partners. We're kind, we're open, we're as patient as possible—with ourself and our spouse—knowing that we both are culpable in causing our train to wobble or crash, whether we were the conductor or the silent observer watching it veer off the tracks.

The good news is that with a little bit of effort there's a new track to be built: a clearer, stronger, more flexible, intimacy-promoting train track that will bring us the peace we've always wanted together. All it takes to get there is a little willingness.

A spending plan for two

I'm going to introduce you to *The Debt-Free Spending Plan*, which I wrote about in detail in my book of the same name. The book offers ways to cut expenses without pain, how to work your money as a couple (even if you have an irregular income), as well as before-and-after examples of how to bring your expenses into balance so you can live without debt or overspending. If you need more specific instruction than I'm offering here, then I urge you to read it.

Here's the basic principle of using a spending plan, which is different than a budget. The word alone—budget—conjures up thoughts of shortage, or belt-tightening, of never having another fulfilled want for the rest of our lives. Many times that's exactly why we resist looking clearly at our finances as a couple: we think that our wants will be relegated to the back corner of the freezer.

A spending plan asks us to *choose* where we want to spend the money we have. If it's the gourmet tea every day over the gym membership, then fine. If it's a monthly massage appointment instead of more entertainment money, then okay. A spending plan is not like a diet, where you're told what you can and can't have. You're the adults. You two are going to make those decisions together for yourselves, with room for each of you to include *wants* as well as needs in your plan.

The only rule that the spending plan imposes is this: *your plan must balance based on what you earn.* Meaning, your spending plan will absolutely keep you living within your means, debt-free, with no additional pressure added to your married life.

The very thought of that—of living within our means—can send a death-ray of panic straight to our heart. But don't worry. The spending plan is a *flexible* tool. There's going to be room for pliability, for moving money around, even for errors.

"Spending proportionally"

What we are going to learn, for the good of our marriage, is the art of *spending proportionally.* What does that mean? It means that we have certain bills and certain daily expenses, as well as the desire for savings and wants, and we need to cover *all* of them. That's right—all of them.

You may be thinking, "Fine, but that's how we got into trouble in the first place—trying to fund *everything we need and want!*" What's different about this spending plan is that you're going to learn to *spend proportionally within the framework of what you earn.* Not above and beyond what you earn, but on the cash you bring home each and every month.

Here's a very basic example. If, after we pay our bills, we have $1,000 a month left to fund our food, fuel, household items, etc., for us both, then we're not going to be in the market for a $275 haircut or four rounds of golf at $325 a month. Am I saying we can never get a decent haircut or play golf? *No.* We need to learn how to allocate our money so we cover *all* of our needs, and some of our wants, too. We may have to get a little creative to do it, and that's exactly what we're going to learn to do.

Will it take some effort at first? Yes. But the good news is that once you put in that initial effort, you'll have your plan forever, and you won't have to reinvent it again unless there are some small adjustments to be made or your income changes, in which case it's simple to re-allocate based on your new earnings.

The skill we're going to learn is what I call "creativity, not credit cards." We're going to learn how to get our basic needs met in affordable ways so we have *more money* for the things we really want. We're going to become accountable—both to ourself and to our marriage.

If this sounds impossible to you, don't panic. Many things seem undoable at the beginning. As Nelson Mandela so eloquently put it, "It is always impossible until it is done."

What if you feel like you're a train wreck with numbers?

One question I'm often asked is: *What if I'm terrible with numbers?*

Let's say that all your life you've gone blank whenever it's time to look at your expenses and see how they balance against your earnings. Perhaps just the *thought* of adding up the total of your monthly bills makes you quake in your boots. If that's you, and/or your partner, don't despair. The spending plan was designed especially for you. It's a five-minutes-a-day plan for people (and couples) who never liked math and need clarity but can never seem to find an easy-enough plan that will work.

Even if you're terrific with numbers, this plan will simplify everything and will help you create a decision-making process in your marriage that's equal and fair.

This plan will greatly aid couples whose preferred method of coping is heads-in-the-sand. It will also help couples in which one partner has been holding the purse strings or has been bearing the brunt of difficult bill-paying and needs to do a better job of sharing the money decisions in their marriage.

The plan will work for *every couple who is willing to use it.* Whether you make $20,000 or $20 million a year, this plan will get you where you need to go: a place of clarity, agreement, and clear decision-making. That's what will take the stress out of your money experiences together, and it's what you need if you want to have a vivid and rich intimate life.

No special skills are needed to work the plan, and no software is required. The only skills you'll need to work this plan are simple addition and a little bit of subtraction. Anyone can do it.

Most of us have not been taught the skills of good and simple money management in marriage—not from our parents, from school, or from any other source—so we must learn it now.

While we're learning this new skill, we need to focus on the positive aspects and refrain from talking-down about our efforts. If we catch ourselves saying something like, "Yeah, we're trying this new thing, but God knows I can never get numbers through my thick head," then stop and regroup. Choose something better to say. We want to speak about this process with respect and willingness for our partner's efforts, for our own efforts, and for our marriage's efforts. Statements such as, "The two of us are trying this new thing that will help us live within our means and will keep the stress out of our marriage. And we're totally willing to learn it."

That will create the foundation for the kind of long-term intimacy and unobstructed sexuality we want to build.

Bills and daily needs

All that's required to balance our monthly spending is addition and subtraction, in a clear and straightforward plan, which the two of us can build together.

We're going to begin by separating our bills from our daily needs. Why do we want to separate what we spend on bills and what we spend on daily expenses? Because our bills are things we *have to pay,* things we get an invoice or mail-in bill for each month; and our daily needs money is a bit more flexible.

Fixed expenses, like mortgage or rent, health insurance, car payments, home or renter's insurance, child care costs, cell phone charges, cable, newspaper subscriptions, gym memberships, and Netflix, show up each and every month.

Some of these bills can be downsized to free up more cash. For instance, ditching the $159-a-month cable bill for a $7.99-a-month movie subscription from Netflix. For now, all we're going to do is list the bills we pay.

Take out a piece of paper or use a plain Word document on the computer and list every bill you both pay, along with the amount due and the monthly due date next to it. If you owe large amounts on credit cards, *don't add up the total you owe.* It will just depress you and make you less willing to try to live within your means. List what you pay monthly, whether it's a bit over the minimum or just the minimum, for each bill, no matter what it is.

If both of you have jobs and you already split up the bills, then list them the way you're currently paying them. Let's use the example of Alexis and Carlos, whose list might begin like this:

Alexis's Bills	Amount	Due Date
Rent	2,200.00	1st
Health insurance	340.16	5th *employee portion for family*

Carlos's Bills	Amount	Due Date
Utilities	88.30	20th

Do this until *all* of the monthly bills—big and small—are listed, including things like newspaper subscriptions, monthly website fees, credit card payments, student loans, anything you owe monthly. Particularly important are bills of a personal nature. For instance, you may have borrowed $40,000 to pay off credit card bills from your parents four years ago and have never tried to pay it back. We don't want any surprises, no "Oh my God, now we owe *that!*" reactions to our spouse when he or she "remembers" a bill or debt. We want to list them all now.

If one spouse earns the money, then separate the bills, about half allotted to each partner to pay. For families with one income, we're going to set it up so that each partner has a separate checking account and some bill-paying responsibility. (We'll talk about why in a moment.)

As much as possible, get monthly accountability for *all* of your bills. This means that if you pay your homeowner's insurance, your car insurance, or other bills quarterly, biannually or annually, *change the schedule to pay for these things monthly.*

Even if it costs you another few dollars each month to set it up that way, do it. Why? Because many of us tend to forget that we have a big car insurance payment coming up in the next month, and we will have to pony up six months' worth of charges for our family. We lose track of the fact that our annual renter's insurance or property taxes are coming up, and we start wringing our hands and snipping at our partner because we never seem to have enough money.

Call the provider and have your payments scheduled on a monthly basis. Do this for any set expense.

With monthly accountability we're going to get a good look at how to live as well as we can on the income we earn, learning to spend proportionally, and then we'll decide what we can reasonably pay back on our debts while we're doing that.

Income

This is the simplest step. Write down earned income on top of the plan, above the list of bills. Remember, *gross* earnings is not the same as net earnings, or what we *clear*. If there's irregular income that doesn't come in year-round, such as earnings from coaching softball or speaking engagements, be sure about what we're clearing and on what timeline we're being paid.

It looks like this:

Carlos's Income	Amount	Pay Date
Bookstore—paid monthly	+897.86	July 1

Alexis's Income	Amount	Pay Date
Marketing Director income	+2392.12	July 3
Marketing Director income	+2392.12	July 17
TOTAL	**+4784.24**	

If you are a partner in a marriage whose income is irregular—for instance, if you're a consultant and can't predict what you will earn—then base your spending plan on what you have in the bank right now and how long you need that money to last. If you have nothing in your checking account, and your family needs your income to live, then you've got to go out and get a job right now.

We cannot engage in what I call "wobbly-legged under-earning," stressing out our family and ourself, because we're consultants or gig-economy workers. If that's your challenge, I strongly recommend that you read the first three chapters in my book, *How to Be an Artist,* which deals with consultants, creatives, entrepreneurs, and artists who have irregular incomes. If you need a day job, then go get one. (The book tells you how to get one that you can live with.) The stress you put on your marriage and intimate life by under-earning will not work to promote the happiness and the intimacy you deserve. Showing up for what you need to show up for will.

I'm stating a rather obvious truism. That is, until our art form or entrepreneurship delivers what we need to live for ourself, our spouse, and our family, we'll need another, regular source of income to create peace in our marriage. My loving suggestion is to not mess around with this truth—to not pretend to be helpless about getting a job. We tank our marriage when we whine, complain, and sit on the sidelines of our earning because we don't feel like being responsible to our marital and family commitments. Under-earning and under-delivering to our marriage means that we erode our partner's trust in us, and that erosion most definitely tears at the fabric of our sex life.

If we need to earn, then we have to show up and do that to preserve our marriage. That's being an adult.

I also believe that one or both spouses have the right to choose lower-paying work that's more meaningful to them in order to create peace in the marriage, to raise a child, or for some other noble venture. When we do that, though, the necessity of living within our means increases dramatically so that we keep stressful money pressure out of our bedroom and out of our family life. We need to be able to live on a downsized spending plan and honor that plan.

Remember our principle of proportional spending? Well, that same guideline applies to earning. If we need to earn to support our partnership and family, then we woman-up or man-up and go out and do just that. Earning when we need to is a commitment to our intimate life, to the peace that will fund the sex life and closeness we're longing for.

Bill-paying should be shared

Many couples who at first glance don't seem to have trouble with money handle it like this: one partner is identified as the better numbers person and manages the finances and pays the bills, while the other partner gets some cash to spend. For lots of marriages, particularly when there's a feeling of having enough money, this system works just fine.

I'm not a big fan of this setup because I don't believe that one partner should be ignorant of what's being paid, how much things cost, and how the amounts of expenses impact the couple's life. But if there's peace in the marriage, no money trouble, and decisions are made together with autonomy being offered to each partner, then it's fine.

In marriages where there has been money trouble, overspending, and vagueness—which is the case for many of us—no one partner should ever be responsible for paying the bills solo. Why? Because when there's financial pressure, overspending, and debt it's *hard* to pay the bills. It's stressful, it's worrisome, and no one spouse should be sweating bullets over paying them while the other partner begs off because he or she is "terrible with finances."

Let me put it bluntly. The claim that we shouldn't have to be a part of the bill-paying because—and this is the real reason—we don't *feel* like it, is a childish excuse that lets the non-bill-paying partner off with no adult responsibility for helping to create agreement within the partnership. Sure, many of us long to be taken care of, but engaging in that stance means we are no longer equal adults, and, subsequently, our sex life suffers. Our partner takes the role of parent while we play the dependent and clueless child, dumping all of the family money angst on our spouse.

Are we really so willing to beg off on our money responsibility when it can cost us equanimity in our sex life?

Couples, whether they have one income or two, need a system for sharing the bill-paying. Here's the simplest thing to do to make sure each partner plays a responsible part in money decisions: each spouse has an individual checking account from which to pay a part of the couple's bills. (I recommend a credit union where you can have multiple accounts for free.)

If both partners bring home a paycheck, create a list of who's paying each bill every month based on when the income comes in. If there's one income, divide up the bills, assigning some bills to each spouse, and transfer some money to the non-earning spouse's account to cover them. We then need to determine the amount each partner needs to cover those bills, as well as daily needs spending (which we'll get into in detail below), to map out our plan.

Once we have our plan mapped out, we will each live on that amount every month. We will pay the bills we're responsible for, deliver to the family the stuff we're in charge of buying as far as daily expenses, and we will also fund our personal needs. Each partner will have accountability, and each will participate in the marital and familial finances.

That's the principle of using a spending plan: to create equality and peace in a marriage.

A quick emotional check-in

Does this sound like a lot of extra work? Does it make you want to scream and rant that you shouldn't have to deal with money at all, and that you don't friggin' want to? Well, join the club. *All* of us who've had money trouble in marriage have felt that way. We want to be taken care of, saved, rescued, and given an E ticket that excuses us from ever having to think about the money responsibilities of adult life.

But here's the thing: by stepping up, by being willing, and by doing our part, even if it's as simple as paying a few bills on time each month, we will rebuild the respect and the *sharing* that's necessary to promote a healthy sex and intimate life in our marriage. We will stop dumping our money troubles and financial decisions on our spouse and become a grown-up partner. Our spouse will respect us more, and we will respect ourself.

Being part of the bill-paying and daily money management represents trustworthiness to our partner, as well as responsibility, caring, willingness, a commitment to clarity, and a giving stance of showing up to share the hard stuff. That right there is a fine basis for building the necessary foundation that supports regular intimacy.

We have to be bigger, more expansive-hearted, and more willing—even in our money managing—if we're going to get to the closeness we really want. To get there, we have to be ready to participate fully in our finances.

Covering our daily needs

Now we've each got ourselves a list of bills and due dates, a notation of what money we're each clearing each month (if we both have jobs), and our paycheck dates. We've separated out a tentative list of who will pay each bill. Now what?

It's time to ballpark our daily needs. In the first few months of using this plan, we'll have to estimate how much we need for daily expenses, and then we'll finesse as we move along. No matter what our ballparked amounts are, we're going to make them balance with our income—that's our charge. Meaning, we absolutely have to create a plan in which what we are paying out is not greater than what we earn.

How do we figure out how much we need for daily things like food and fuel, drug store items, personal care, postage, dry cleaning, etc., without digging up our past spending history? We guesstimate. Most of us who have had money trouble spend erratically, so digging up past bank statements is often less accurate than simple guesswork. We may have spent $350 at Costco last month and don't even remember what we purchased, so that's not going to help us understand what we *actually* have to spend for our needs.

We want clarity based on what we have now. Not what we were once spending, but the actual amount of cash we have to live on. Once more: it's not how much we *want* to spend, but how much we actually *have* that will determine our plan and create peace in our marriage.

We're going to line out about twelve to fifteen categories for our daily needs—no more—and we're going to use them to fund our daily expenses. Why use only twelve to fifteen categories? Because we want to be able to keep track of this thing in five minutes a day. We want to keep it short and sweet, simple and easy, so we can keep our head, heart, and willingness in doing it. We don't want to check out after a month because the damn thing is too complicated or it consumes too much of our mental or emotional bandwidth. We want a *shortcut* to keeping our spending clear.

Not only do we need this thing to be simple if it's ever going to work, but we also need it to work right off the bat in our marriage—not six months from now, not next year. We need it *now.* Keeping it short and sweet means we can learn it quickly and make it work for us the very first month of using it.

Let's look at daily needs using the example of Carlos and Alexis. Carlos works at home as a writer and a handful of hours as part-time bookstore employee. He's also the primary caretaker for the couple's four-year-old daughter, so he can reasonably wear jeans to work every day. His daily costs for clothing will not be as high as Alexis's, who works as a marketing director at a hospital where there's a professional dress code.

When we sit down to talk about the amounts that fund our daily needs, the object is to be fair and reasonable. We want to divide up the duties (and the money attached to each) based on what each partner reasonably needs to cover, and what each is contributing in terms of labor to family life. For instance, if Carlos is most often the partner who takes the couple's four-year-old daughter to the doctor for her allergy shots, then he will need to manage the child's co-pay money in his plan.

We make the plan work for our specific needs—for the way we divide up labor for the family, and the special needs that come up. Here's two more examples: if Alexis's father is ill and she needs to drive their car two hours to go visit him every week, then she and Carlos need to add that fuel money to her plan. If Carlos has back issues from sitting still for hours at the computer, coupled with lifting up their daughter all day long, and massage is the only thing that relieves his pain, then the couple needs to include a reasonable amount to cover those costs in his plan.

Let's talk about spending categories

We're going to use Carlos and Alexis as our example couple. We'll list each partner's individual spending plan, with some bill-paying assigned to each spouse.

Carlos and Alexis split up the money for food. He buys meat, fish, and produce at the local market each week. His wife is responsible for buying cheese, eggs, wine, cereal, basic food stuffs, and some household items at the local Trader Joe's. When they are constructing their plans, the couple will need to guesstimate just how much they each will need to cover those items for their family. Note that some daily needs in Carlos's plan will be personal, and others will serve the family unit.

Here's Carlos's daily needs list for the month:

Carlos Daily Needs	Amount
Food (meat, fish, produce)	225.00
Fuel	95.00
Household	30.00
Haircut (including tip)	45.00
Drug store	25.00
Postage	10.00
Dry cleaning	25.00
Clothing	35.00
Daughter's clothes	30.00
Daughter's co-pays	35.00
Carlos's co-pays	35.00
Monthly massage	55.00
Entertainment for family	200.00
Date money	60.00
Extra	25.00
TOTAL	**-930.00**

Let's take a look at a few things on Carlos's list. First, he reasonably covers the things he needs to deliver to his marriage and family: food (groceries), some household items, his daughter's clothing and medical co-pays, family entertainment, and some romantic date money to take his wife out. Then there are things he needs personally: drug store items, dry cleaning, medical co-pays, monthly massage, and postage money. He's also got a bit of cash that he labels "extra" for picking up a pizza when he and Alexis don't feel like cooking, or to buy something he wants for himself. Alexis will make out her daily needs list for herself.

Note that the money to cover these expenses is *allocated to each spouse at the beginning of the month based on what each partner is responsible for.* Once it's allocated, it's his or hers to manage as he or she sees fit, as long as what's needed for family life is delivered.

We don't micromanage how our partner spends what's been allocated, and we don't take back the assignment that each has been given. For instance, Alexis doesn't get to say, "Hey, babe, I need another thirty dollars; you can take it out of our daughter's clothing allotment." That's not going to fly. We build respect for one another by being responsible for the expenses we agreed to manage.

We don't tank the amounts in our plan in the first week and then expect our spouse to bail us out. We don't go crazy at Costco and then call up our partner and bawl him or her out for not earning enough. We simply live within the categories we set out, month by month, learning as we go to live with the allotted amount.

When we're responsible to our marriage within the framework of the spending plan we build trust. And we know now what trust builds, right? Yep. You've got it. It builds intimacy.

How do you use this thing anyway?

Let's say we've each got our list of bills, we've each got a ballpark list of daily needs, and we've listed what we clear in earnings every month. Now what? Those of us who spend vaguely and without any concern for how much we have each month are not going stop spending just because we wrote this thing down. We need something stronger than that to get us some genuine daily clarity!

Here's the simplicity of how this works. Once we allocate our daily needs spending for the month, we're going to use a tool I call *The Magic Little Notebook* to keep track of our daily spending. This is where the rubber meets the road in changing our behavior; it's also where lots of people step right off the train and sink right back into the mud. Keep your head in. It's simple, and can help save our marriage.

Having a list of what we're *supposed to be spending* each month won't help at all if we wait to see what we've spent *after* we've already spent it. This is the crazy-obvious point about why tools like Quicken and Quickbooks don't help those of us who have issues with money. We need something that helps us know what we have to spend *before we spend it.*

The whole point of the spending plan is to *look before we spend.* We don't spend one damn dime unless we have it. *That's* how we live within the cash income we have, and it's how we build respect for each other in our marriage with money.

Here's how it works: First, get an inexpensive three-by-five-inch notebook at the drugstore or use your Notes app on your phone. Write down all of the items on your daily needs list, one on each page. Here's an example with a modest income:

On one page:

Food for July   +325.00

7/6 Lucky's market   -68.33

                                        +256.67 (balance)

7/15 Dean's Produce   -42.00

                                        +214.67 (balance)

On another page:

Household for July   +30.00

7/7 Target—kitchen stuff   -18.22

                                        +11.78 (balance)

The Magic Little Notebook is designed to help keep us on track when we're out in the world spending. This simple system is the antidote to the crazy-making of the joint checking account approach, where neither partner knows if the other is spending money.

This makes it easy to *always look before you spend.*

This means that if I'm heading to the grocery store at the beginning of the month I can't blow my monthly grocery allotment of $325 in the first week. I've got to parse it out *reasonably* (e.g., $325 divided by four weeks is $81.25; if there are five weeks, then it's $65.00 per week). This is how we stay within our allotted amounts. For things like personal care, beauty products, household items, etc., we can easily shop *once a month* for those items, so it's easier to keep track of what we have to spend.

I recommend having an "extra" category with twenty-five to fifty dollars allotted for it, because life's little emergencies will always show up, and we want to be able to cover them when they do.

What to do if you go over

Let's say you're using this simple system and you go to the dry cleaners and your bill is $35, but you've only got $30 set aside for dry cleaning category. Do you have to leave your clothes there until next month? No. You can move money around from category to category based on your monthly needs.

For example, you might look in your household category and ask yourself, "Do we have everything we need for the house already? Saran wrap, toilet paper, laundry soap?" If so, then move five dollars into your dry cleaning category and pick up your clothes. The notes in your Magic Little Notebook will look like this:

Dry Cleaners	30.00
9/10 Stella's Cleaners	-35.00
	-5.00
9/10 Moved from Household	+5.00
	0.00

Household	30.00
9/7 Target—kitchen stuff	-18.22
	+1.78
9/10 Move to Cleaner	-5.00
	+6.78

Always write down any time you move money from one category to another, even if it seems high-maintenance. Why? Because you need to know just how much is in each category before you spend. Also, if we note that we're going over in one daily needs category all the time, that means we need to adjust our plan a bit to cover the need.

For "hoarders" who love to stock up, or those who take all of your clothes to the dry cleaners three times a year for a charge of $300 or more a pop, guess what? You're going to have to learn a new way. The way to live within your means and be accountable in your marriage is to only purchase what you need *for right now*—for this week or this month. Don't stock up. For those of us who have a lack of money clarity, stocking up is usually code for "debting," meaning we get a thrill out of spending because it's "a good deal," but we are doing so by debting against our other expenses. This won't work.

Most of us want to argue the point that when the bulk warehouse has a special on a package of twenty-five pairs of socks, or a pack of forty pork chops for fifty-five dollars, that we have to scoop up the deal because it's a "money saver." That's just not true. If I spend fifty-five dollars on pork chops from my seventy dollars a week for my part of the groceries, I've just blown more than half of my food money, and I still need produce, eggs, milk, etc. I may argue that the deal weighs in heavily for buying the meat, but are we really going to eat pork chops every night this month? Not likely. Do I really need twenty-five pairs of new socks in one fell swoop? Hardly.

Unless I have ten children, buying in bulk is a smokescreen for overspending. I'll say that again. Unless I have a very large family, there is no need to buy a huge quantity of anything.

Buy what you need, week by week, and I promise you it will be less than you think. Live within the amounts you set out, using your notebook to remain accountable.

Does this feel like it will be impossible to manage? Are you freaking out over the careful way you'll have to spend to make this work? Good. That's normal. We all feel that way when we begin. But we are not doing this so we can be good little money citizens. We are learning to live within our means so we can have more of the important stuff that we really want in the world—and in our marriage.

We're talking about more entertainment money, more vacation money, more money for romance and fun. More cash for the things we love like clothes, art supplies, a trek through Spain, or a groovy music camp for our child. Living within set amounts for our daily needs translates directly to more fun and less focus on bills, debt, and expenses.

Want money for a new computer? Want money for tennis lessons? Want to try painting and need to buy supplies? Want to take a yoga seminar? Then you're going to need the clarity of living within your daily needs to free up that cash to fund your wants.

That's the magic of this thing. We learn to live simply in our daily needs categories so we can be accountable to our marriage, surely, but also so we can have more cash for the things we want in life. That's the principle.

When we create that kind of accountability, we not only begin to have more ease and delight with each other, we also create the peace in our marriage that leads to an unobstructed intimate life.

And that's the whole ballgame.

Face-front with two spending plans

Here's a look at a full couple's spending plan with each spouse's part accounted for. Let's use Carlos and Alexis as an example:

CARLOS'S SPENDING PLAN

Income	Amount	Pay Date
Bookstore (paid monthly)	+897.86	July 1st
TOTAL	**+897.86**	

Bills	Amount	Due Date
Utilities	88.30	20th
Car insurance	89.32	8th
Netflix	7.99	6th
TOTAL	**-185.61**	

Daily Needs for July	Amount
Food (meat, fish, produce)	225.00
Fuel	95.00
Household	30.00
Haircut (including tip)	45.00
Drug store	25.00
Postage	10.00
Dry cleaning	25.00
Clothing	35.00
Daughter's clothes	30.00
Daughter's copays	35.00
Copays-Carlos	35.00
Monthly massage	55.00
Entertainment for family	200.00
Date money	60.00
Extra	25.00
TOTAL	**-930.00**

Carlos's Total Monthly Expenses	-1,115.61
Total Income	+897.86
Balance	-217.75
Check from Alexis	+217.75

ALEXIS'S SPENDING PLAN

Income	Amount	Pay Date
Hospital	2,392.12	July 3rd
Hospital	2,392.12	July 17th
TOTAL	**4,784.24**	

Bills	Amount	Due Date
To Carlos from first check	217.75	1st
Rent	2,200.00	1st
Health insurance for family	340.16	5th *(employee portion)*
Renter's insurance	19.91	10th
Cell phones	189.60	10th
Credit card	140.00	15th
TOTAL	**3,107.42**	

Daily Needs	Amount
Groceries/house	300.00
Transportation	125.00
Household	30.00
Haircut (including tip)	20.00
Drug store	45.00
Postage	10.00
Coffee bar	35.00
Lunches out	50.00
Dry cleaning	55.00
Clothing	85.00
Copays	35.00
Extra	25.00
TOTAL	**815.00**

Alexis's Total Monthly Expenses	-3,922.42	
Total Income	+4,784.24	
Balance	+861.82 *(additional cash directed to savings)*	

Savings	+861.82
Vacation	200.00
Healthy reserve	130.00
Short-term savings	100.00

College fund	100.00
Car repairs	85.00
New TV fund	65.00
Down payment fund	181.82
TOTAL	**861.82**

Let's note a few things about Carlos's and Alexis's full spending plans. Given that Carlos does the larger share of the child care and works in a bookstore part time, his income is lower than Alexis's—a choice the couple made to both fund his writing projects and support their daughter. But since the couple chooses to have Carlos coordinate more of the family needs than his salary allows, they need to augment his plan by $217.75 from Alexis's first-of-the-month check.

This setup is what works best for them as a couple, so each would be responsible for some bills and daily needs, and so the numbers would fit with the way they divide labor in their family life. Craft your plan however it works best for your marriage, as long as both partners have bill-paying responsibility and daily needs accountability.

To free up more cash, Carlos and Alexis decided to get rid of cable in favor of an inexpensive streaming service, got rid of their home phone, and sold their newer car (payments were more than five hundred dollars per month). They kept their eight-year-old car, which was running fine and had been well taken care of. Since the car was out of warranty, they began setting aside eighty-five dollars a month in an account for car repairs. (This is a must for any couple driving used cars.)

After those simple changes, they applied some easy creativity to living within their daily needs amounts. Carlos discovered a hip Greek produce shop in their neighborhood that charges 30 percent less for fruits and vegetables, and he now walks there with their daughter. Alexis goes to the beauty school for $10 haircuts (including tip) and allows a few extra bucks for a blow dry there.

Alexis gives herself $35 a month for the coffee bar and $50 for lunches out, and the other days she brings her lunch and has coffee at home. She gave up expensive makeup, cleansers, etc., in favor of lower-cost products she gets at the drugstore.

The couple juggles childcare when Carlos is working, particularly on weekend days, but when they can't cover it, Alexis's folks babysit their daughter, saving them at least five hundred dollars a month.

Carlos handles fewer bills, but manages more of the daily needs money, including the couples' entertainment and date money, because it makes his wife feel more romantic if he picks up the check when they go out.

By making these simple changes and adapting the plan to their own specific needs and wants, Alexis and Carlos were able to free up more than eight hundred dollars a month for savings and for things they really want. They stopped running up debt every month, and after three months of using their plans they cut up their credit cards, consolidated all their debt on one low-interest card, and agreed to pay 20 percent over the minimum each month until it's paid off. When Carlos gets paid for a writing gig, which is usually about every three months, they use the "windfall money" rule for nonrecurring additional cash: one-third to debt, one-third to savings, and one-third to something they really want.

They live only on their earned income now, and though their relationship had not been plagued by awful fights about money, it had been full of tension, worry, and stress, and the pressure of their debt had been mounting and negatively affected their intimacy. Once they had used their plan for a solid two months, they reported feeling freer, lighter, and more in love.

Though it doesn't seem like it would be such a direct line from creating money clarity to having unobstructed intimacy—particularly when we're in a standoff or shutdown with our partner—couples report over and over again that it does work that way. When we have both an agreement and a plan, we respect each other more, we're easier with each other, we're more content in our family situation, and because we're beginning to stash money for the things we want and need, *we relax in our hearts.*

With a relaxed heart, we're able to look over and see the good in our partner—the charm, the grace, the delightful quirks, the sweetness and the strength. That's all the stuff we need to lead us back to desire, back to the easy-on-the-soul sex and intimacy that we so want and crave.

How the plan keeps you from micromanaging each other

There's another angle on our historical money vagueness and over-spending that can harm our marriage. When we have no clarity, we often end up micromanaging each other's spending.

Many couples who have financial trouble favor the joint-account, no-one-ever-writes-anything-down-in-the-checkbook approach. We wander out shopping, buying without clarity, and praying our partner isn't spending. When we find out that he or she is spending randomly just like we are, we end up fighting about it.

So, how do we get out of the madness of micromanaging each other about spending? Here's how: we create and maintain a personal spending plan for both partners that provides clarity *before* we spend.

If my husband has paid his part of the bills and delivered the necessary household items from his plan and has some leftover cash at the end of the month, *then he can spend it on whatever he damn well pleases.* The same is true for me; for instance, if I have forty dollars extra in fuel money because I chose to cycle to work one week and I want to buy a blouse with it, that's my business. Once we allocate our monthly money, it's each partner's prerogative to manage it as he or she sees fit—as long as what's been assigned is being delivered to the marriage and the family—so we can back off and offer our partner some breathing room.

This simple side benefit of the plan can put a marriage that's been plagued by money micromanaging (and the resulting fights) back on a respect-each-other trajectory.

And we must have that respect if we're ever going to be able to get naked with each other on a regular basis.

Savings saves you

When my husband and I were in downward spirals of financial distress (which was most of our first marriage) people would always ask us if we saved money. And my response was always the same: "We can't save money; we've got too much debt."

Personally, I also had a weird relationship to savings accounts. The few times I had them, I would either use my savings money as a slush fund for overspending when I was shopping, or I'd be terrified to touch the cash. What I've discovered while coaching couples over the past twelve years is that this response is fairly common. When we're inexperienced at saving, and more experienced at overspending and running up debt, we often zone out on how to wisely use our savings if it's all in one account.

Here's how we can handle that.

My husband and I use what I call a Multiple Savings Account approach. We have multiple accounts at a credit union (where there are no service charges at all) nicknamed for specific things. For instance, we have a Couples Reserve in case one of us loses our job. Then, we each have individual Short-Term Savings accounts to use in emergencies instead of using credit cards. We also have savings accounts for car repairs, health care (for expenses not covered by insurance), and rent increases. There's also an account to cover the sales tax I get when I sell my books, art, and music.

We also have accounts for our wants, both as a couple and as individuals: travel, new computer, Christmas, art for the house, and more. When we have a need or want that's unaddressed—costs to promote one of my books, a trip with friends for my husband—we create an account and *save* for the thing we want, adding a bit of money to it each month or allocating money if we get a bonus or an extra bit of cash.

The idea of multiple savings accounts is to cover *all* of our genuine needs and some of our wants so we can ease up mentally and emotionally. We begin to understand that there's room in our marriage for each of us to have the things we want individually, as well as the things we want as a couple.

There's a consciousness to this savings thing, and when we begin to employ it, it makes us feel lighter about our money, even if we're only saving a few bucks every month in each savings account.

When there's ease and lightness in our relationship to our money, we feel that we're taking good care of our marriage and each other, which allows us to move toward each other sensually in an effortless way. Our intimacy flows without any obstacles, and we get to experience the joy of our marriage—sweetly, amorously, and certainly sexually.

A bill-paying plan for two

Now that you've mapped out your spending plan you need to know *when* to pay each bill. You can't just pay everything as it comes in or you won't have enough money for your daily needs expenses the way they're mapped out in your plan. You have to have a timeline for paying your bills based on when cash comes in so you can cover your daily and weekly needs like food and fuel.

If you receive a monthly paycheck, like Carlos, it's pretty easy. When you get your check, you'll pay your assigned bills, put the allocated money into savings accounts, and then fund your daily needs from your checking account based on your spending plan. If you get paid weekly or every other week, the way Alexis does, then you need a bill-paying schedule, with each bill assigned to a particular paycheck.

If you need help with this step, please consult chapters three and four in my book, *The Debt-Free Spending Plan,* which detail exactly how to set it up and use a bill-paying plan. The object is to know *exactly* when we're paying each bill, and *exactly* how much we have to spend on daily needs, so we always have clarity and don't overspend.

These are the pieces of the plan: clarity in our bill-paying, a little notebook for daily needs that we consult before we spend, and a mapped-out approach to saving for what we need and want. It's that simple.

As any couple who's been through the dark tunnel of money disasters and come out on the other side into the cool, crisp air of financial clarity and renewed intimacy can tell you, this little plan, practiced for just a few minutes a day, is worth its weight in gold.

What do you get out of this?

Most couples' will respond to this system with one (or more) of the following responses: "Are you kidding? You actually think we should write down everything we spend and look to see if we have the cash before we spend it?" Or, "You want us to live week to week and month to month without stocking up *and* cut some expenses too?" Or, "You expect us to *save?* On our income?" The answer to all of these is, *yes.* Here's why.

When we stop engaging in mindless spending and get clarity on what we have to spend, something revolutionary happens: *we get to keep the money we set aside for our wants.*

This is the root of this plan: the freedom to have our individual wants and needs, as well as having wants and needs as a couple, while living within our means. It helps us get out of the cycle of always *paying* and instead, helps us begin *living.*

When I used to go crazy with my cash and credit cards, I valued the addictive jones of vague overspending over the things I wanted, like a weekend away, money for my art supplies, a new computer for my husband, etc. I had to realize that *every mindless dime I spent was literally stealing money from the things I really wanted.*

My husband and I now fund the things we love—dining out, date nights, clothing, vacations, holiday money, projects that are meaningful to our hearts and souls—even if the amounts we set aside are modest.

That's the power of the marital spending plan: we get monthly bills accountability, fund our daily needs, spend within our allotted amounts, save a bit, *and* we fund our wants, too, so our life is about *living* and engaging in what we love together, not about just getting by.

Think about that for a moment. Think how that will help promote your marriage's intimacy, closeness, and joy with each other. Money clarity—and the ease that comes with it—really is a direct line to greater closeness and amorousness because it makes us feel *relieved* that we're covering what we need to cover, *and* we're addressing our wants. It also makes us feel responsible—to each other and to ourself—and the respect that's built by that clarity gives us access to each other's hearts, bodies, and spirits, with no obstacles in the way.

If that sounds amazing to you, I'm telling you now that it's well within your grasp. All it takes to halt the rollicking machine of overspending and money pressure in your marriage is to craft a simple spending plan and—here's the key—use it. Then sit back with your partner and watch as the whole landscape of your marriage grows greener and more lush.

A big idea, but a bigger payoff

The Naked Money theme is a big idea in a book about marital intimacy. In truth, I can't do justice to the full implementation of the plan in one chapter, so if you've had money and debt trouble in your marriage, I lovingly suggest that you read *The Debt-Free Spending Plan,* chapters one through four, on how to create a plan, and chapters seven and nine on couples. That bit of reading will give you a more solid foundation to create peace in your marriage with your finances.

As we wrap up this chapter, I'd like to talk about the payoff for the effort I'm encouraging. Money, as we said before, and having trouble with it, will tank our intimate life faster than anything else in marriage. It will drain us, piss us off, make us feel trapped, and wring every bit of desire we ever had for our partner out of our bodies and souls. It will kill our sex life. That's just what money trouble does.

The payoff for detailing how we're going to manage the finances in our marriage is this: *we get our intimate life back.* If we truly want a regular, close, and even voluptuous intimate life, then we've got to get a practical handle on this monkey—to release the grip of its straining fingers and toss it off our backs and out of our souls. A couple's spending plan creates the peace that we've been longing for, the agreement that we need, and the opening into respect that fuels a rich and fulfilling sensual life.

Remember, to change the landscape of our money life, and thus our intimacy, we need to take *action.* That doesn't mean just talking about it, digging up our history, "processing" the issues or (worse) ignoring them altogether. The good news is, we now have a guide—a set of suggestions—that can bring clarity to our marriage's money *in one short month.*

This work, as challenging as it may seem at the beginning, is the bedrock for what will come to our marriage as a result of doing it: free-flowing warmth, respect, willingness, desire, amorousness, and closeness.

The perfect foundation on which to build a regular, sensual, and sexual intimate life.

Rory and LeeAnn

When I was first asked by Rory and LeeAnn to coach them on their intimacy, lifestyle, and money issues, I realized they had a challenge most of us aren't faced with. Their earnings were way higher than their bills and needs. Their houses and new cars were paid for. They had plenty of money for luxuries. And since they didn't have kids, they had no upcoming large-scale expenses, like college tuition or kids' weddings. That said, they still had money issues, fueled by a spend-what-you-make perception of believing they would always have the same large-scale income coming in.

In our first meeting, it was clear that they both loved each other and even enjoyed each other, yet their overspending—they were spending everything they earned, and even running up a bit of debt—was causing trouble in their marriage and intimate life. They each had a huge sense of guilt about their money choices.

Rory was upset with LeeAnn for spending thousands on couture clothing, personal trainers, and body therapies, as well as for funding a small business that was costing them well over three hundred thousand dollars a year and wasn't profitable. When they traveled, she insisted they patronize the most expensive hotels and restaurants. LeeAnn was angry at Rory for spending hundreds of thousands on multiple country club memberships, a vintage car collection, and particularly for "being a sap," as she put it, paying off large-scale debt for family members who would be back at their door a few years later with another pay-off request. He also insisted on picking up the check whenever they went out with friends, no matter how expensive the tab.

Both partners knew their anger and irritation were keeping them from having sex as often as they'd like, and, in Rory's words, they "avoided each other at opposite ends of the house a lot."

"Our house is too big for us anyway, so if we want to avoid talking to each other, we can disappear on each other for days," LeeAnn added.

I shared what I know about couples and money. First, that overspending is a *process addiction*, meaning it has nothing to do with how much money we have. Instead, it has to do with a ramped-up need to feel taken care of. We spend intensely to make ourselves feel like we "have enough." We think it will create a feeling of safety, but the pressure only leads to a sensation of sinking sand in our marriages, producing desperation instead of ease, which then affects our intimacy.

When we talked about what was at the root of their need to overspend and "live too high," as Rory put it,

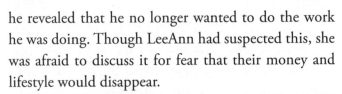

he revealed that he no longer wanted to do the work he was doing. Though LeeAnn had suspected this, she was afraid to discuss it for fear that their money and lifestyle would disappear.

LeeAnn said, "I feel like we're overspending to fulfill some kind of gratification that we're not giving each other."

The problem with spending this way, I told them, is that the meal or the vacation we're paying for *always ends*, and what we're really searching for is an intimacy that endures and won't end.

Our approach was simple: we first created a couple's spending plan (as detailed in this chapter), so LeeAnn and Rory could both see what money they had, what they really needed, and where they could cut out unnecessary spending and still feel well taken care of, and even have some of their luxuries accounted for.

Then we had the harder conversation: Rory needed out of his high-pressure human resources company. He had helped to build it over a number of years, and though it was a huge success, he was exhausted. "I'm done—that's the truth I haven't been telling my wife," he told me. "I'm not sleeping, I can't digest my food, and my hair is falling out in clumps."

LeeAnn laughed at this last item, and said, "Isn't that what happens at fifty-seven?" When she saw his eyes start to water, she got it.

Since we had already established clarity in their finances, it became clear that Rory could reasonably quit working and, with a few downsizing choices, they would be able to live perfectly well for years without worry. I asked Rory how it would feel to set an end date for leaving his job, and the tension visibly left his face and shoulders; his answer was clear. I asked LeeAnn what it would mean for her, and if she understood her husband's need to stop. "I do," she said. "But I'm afraid of the changes."

As soon as we dove in to the real issue behind their overspending, and the resulting ding to their intimacy, their choices became much easier for the two of them. Rory gave a six-month notice at his job. LeeAnn admitted that she never really liked their huge house and would prefer to live in a smaller community where they could "hang out and be close" in a nice, but more modest, house. "I'd like to be able to shout across the house and have him hear me," she admitted.

They agreed to begin practicing the communication techniques in this book, checking in each week about how they felt about the changes they were making, and agreed to try the Naked Date. They stopped paying off family members' debts, stopped joining multiple country clubs, and modified their daily and monthly spending.

Six months later, Rory had left his job, the couple sold their large house and two rental units and moved to the lake town LeeAnn had her eye on. Rory began teaching poetry at the local arts center—an art form he had left behind years ago—and LeeAnn got involved in a local green organization, working on environmental issues.

When I asked how their intimate life had changed, Rory said, "One word: *miracle*. You could say it was retirement that did it, but it wasn't that. It was telling the truth, learning how to talk to each other in small chunks of time, prioritizing what we really want."

LeeAnn said, "I have a lover again. I didn't even know what I was missing."

When I queried them about what they learned that stood out for their future life together, LeeAnn said, "You can't put a price on love. You've got to make choices together that let you both feel it and live it."

CHAPTER SEVEN
NAKED JOY AND HAPPINESS

Marriage and desire

My husband has edited two short story anthologies—one on marriage and one on desire. At a dinner party where the topics of these books were mentioned, a man at the table said casually, "Desire and marriage? Those seem like two mutually exclusive topics." Although the line got a good laugh, it was a sad and sorry commentary on modern marriage and the lack of fulfillment it often offers us.

That's why I wrote this book. Why should marriage and desire be mutually exclusive? Why are we not getting the joy out of our marriages that we should be getting? We know we love each other, so why should a dulling down of our sexual life be the expected result of being committed to each other over time?

I don't believe—and no one is going to convince me—that drifting is the intent of marriage.

Closeness is its intent—walking together through life's good, bad, and overwhelming experiences with love at our center, with the amorous glue of devotion and passion holding us up, reminding us why it is good to be alive and to be alive *together*.

We can't expect that our long-term loving will look and feel like it did when we were dating or newly married. Marriage is different than dating or early love. It asks for more than our one-on-one desire for each other. But there is a realm of mature experience in intimacy that's just waiting for us to claim it, as long as we have even a little bit of willingness to try.

If we want to experience the full-on nature of our love, we have to find ways to *practice* it which don't consume our life or require major archeological digging into our psychology to get there.

We need shortcuts and easy strategies that will work within the framework of our busy, often crazily scheduled, stressful lives. We need a few *right quick* ways to get to our intimacy—our affection, romance, sex, sensuality, communication, and lifestyle and money agreements—so we have unobstructed access to each other's hearts, souls, and bodies.

Choose intimacy

Close and fulfilling intimacy over the course of a marriage is not a myth. It's not even hard to master. All it takes is a bit of effort and the commitment to apply a few easily learned skills.

We have the power to interrupt the voices in our head (as well as from our culture) that say marriage will dull itself over time. We can use whatever tools we can get our hands on to open up our body and spirit to a meaningful love experience—a regular practice of owning and holding it, feeling it, and delighting in it.

When we're willing to *practice loving*, we get to have a deepening of our amorousness and a heightening of our sexual connection with our spouse over the course of years. By having a practice of love, we get a marriage filled with fulfilment.

The blessing of a long and happy marriage is the longevity of our closeness, the prowess of our constantly renewing sensuality, our ability to communicate, our practiced ways of creating agreement in our choices. All of these things deepen our growth together, making our

NAKED JOY AND HAPPINESS

marriage strong and rich. Straight-up, these things fire our desire over time. There's nothing else in the whole wide world like having a lover who has our back, who knows us, shows us devotion and willingness, offers us fiery desire, and walks with us year in and year out, loving us the whole way. Nothing else comes close.

Most of us who are married say we want to feel like we're in love. We want our marriage to be more than just a base from which to craft the external shape of a married life. We'd like it to be passionate and fun—an experience of devotion, exploration, and intimate delights.

We know that it also has to be a rock we can stand upon to weather the troubling, stressful, and sometimes grievous things life throws at us. We need that loyalty and that security in our commitment.

Most of us already have that loyalty and a secure bond. What we may be missing is the sweet stuff: the continuing intimacy that makes us feel like we're in love and the sexy stuff that brings us the delight we so crave with our partner.

Intimacy is a choice we make. It is an adult experience based upon a deepening, an exploration, and a willingness to keep exploring.

This book's strategies are guidelines for *choosing intimacy* in our marriage. By practicing the Naked Marriage tips offered here, we're declaring our commitment before the altar of love. With our actions, we're communicating that we mean to love our partner as well as we can, that we intend to have a *lifelong love affair*: a marriage filled with love and sex, joy and happiness. That's hugely powerful.

We are partners in love

We all know that it's naïve to think that sex and sensuality are one-way roads to happiness in a marriage. It's also naïve to pretend that we can omit sensual intimacy—sidestepping it for more platonic forms of existing together—and still have a fulfilling, happy experience in our loving. We were never meant to be roommates, never meant to have a duty-bound, obligatory relationship with our chosen partner.

Though it's obvious that I'm a huge fan of the Naked Marriage, my premise is based on a much broader idea than having a weekly sexual experience or sitting down to talk. The broader theme is that we can learn to be naked in all of the things that lead to an open and fulfilling marital life. Openness in our affection, romance, sex, communication, money agreement—all of it—fuels more love and a deepening of our experience together.

We are partners in love. That is our place with each other, the role we have chosen by marrying one another. So it behooves us to find ways to get to that loving. We need to express it, practice it, and feel it physically, spiritually, emotionally, and sexually.

We all understand what it was like to be loved (or not loved) as a child. We know what it felt like to be paid attention to or ignored, to be considered and guided or shunted to the side. We know whether our parents included our emotional needs in their consideration of us, whether they allowed room for us to have wants or feelings of our own. We remember whether they were affectionate with us verbally and physically, whether they laughed with us and delighted in us or marginalized, bullied, or demeaned us. They are so visceral, we may remember those experiences as if they happened yesterday. And so it is in marriage. The feelings run just as deep, reverberating just as earth-shaking and profound.

Those childhood experiences live on inside us in a primal way, and we can take a valuable lesson from how we still feel about them as adults. They can be the guiding principle of how we learn to cherish our marital partner now—how we behave with our spouse in our efforts to be close. We want to understand the depth and the reverberations of what we have undertaken in agreeing to love our partner in marriage for a lifetime.

It is a very primal thing indeed to be loved. To be held dear, to be treated with gentleness and kindness, to be considered and included, to walk with our partner's heart inside our own. Then, from that love and consideration, to be included in our partner's time, efforts, and willingness to please—meaning, to be desired and pursued, offered heat and longing, and to know that our partner cherishes and even adores us.

We want to do more than know we love each other; we want to *feel* it.

And here's the truth that's underlying all of the efforts we've talked about, the theme of *Naked Marriage*: if we want a devoted love affair, then we have to show up for it. We have to make an effort. We have to have a *practice* of love.

We don't get a pass because we're busy; we don't get a leave of absence because there's trouble; there are no sick days. Loving is a lifelong, full-time job. Our efforts to love our partner matter.

We won't be remembered for meeting deadlines or landing that big deal; we will be remembered for how well we loved. When we bring joy to our partner and our marriage, we not only ease the load of our spouse and our family, we also help our own heart, and our partner's heart, feel what is truly important in life.

When we love well, we delight in the sweetness of living. We are held dear in our older years, pined over and adored for how well we gave the gifts of our love, our body, our desire, our devotion, and our spirit.

And who among us doesn't want that?

Take what you like

I want you to view this book as a take-what-what-you-like-and-leave-the-rest offering—suggestions and guideposts from my own personal experience (as well as from lessons learned from my couples' coaching and interviewing) to implement or not as you see fit in your own marriage. It's a collection of things to try. If they resonate with you and make your heart rumble a bit, then I urge you to keep using them to enhance your loving.

What's important is to recognize that life will not support a fulfilling intimate life without your commitment. *You* have to claim it, and you have to find ways to do that on a regular basis.

My message is about being willing to do just that. It's about finding the shortcuts to intimacy—the things that, done with regularity, will get you there in short and sweet time intervals. It is the antidote to drifting and an offering of strategies that help us build prowess in our loving over the course of our whole marriage.

If our loving is the one thing we will most remember when we pass from this life, then why should we not claim the love that matters to us? It's ours to claim, and we should claim it. That's the point of *Naked Marriage*.

The timelessness of love

Previously, I mentioned that when my mother-in-law was in her eighties, long after her husband had died, she had a love affair with a man who was two years younger. She went through all of the stuff we all do when we fall in love: delight, joy, giddiness, angst at separation, fights about how to work things out and find commitment. At the beginning of their relationship, my husband and I would get a call every two months or so from her partner saying goodbye to us because, as he'd say, "We've had a fight and it's surely *over*." (They'd be back together within three days every time, as if nothing had happened.)

What weighed on them differently from those of us who are in the early or middle years of adulthood and marriage is *time*.

When we're thirty and we're drifting from each other, or in our mid-forties being bowled over by the responsibilities of married life, or in our fifties having gotten used to distancing, we don't think much about our mortality. It feels like there are years ahead to patch things up, to get back on the right track emotionally. We defer dealing with our drifting and distancing until the kids are older, the job deadlines are fielded, the communication breakdowns have faded in importance, or the long hours at work or the money trouble that's plaguing us has somehow become part of the woodwork. We think we can live with chasms between us and drift, because we believe there are years stretched out in front of us to find our way back again.

Ask anyone who's over sixty-five and they will tell you that it all goes by in a blink. *Here and now matters.* Whether we're showing up and sharing our love now matters.

Of the couples I spoke with while writing this book who stayed close over the course of years, several spoke about something rather profound: warding off mortality by staying intimately connected—by building, a little bit each week, a kind of timelessness into their lives by being sexual and intimate.

Though time is ticking by, their constant has been each other—an offering of desire that still lifts them spiritually and has begun to stand outside of time. It's the gift of having a practice of love: a way to stop the world from spinning and disappear into something higher and sweeter that can connect them to what transcends.

The truth is, each touch and each kiss brings us closer to the *last kiss* and the *last caress.* Seen through that lens, it makes each intimate experience richer and more meaningful. As one husband said to me, "I couldn't have known how rich it was going to feel years later that we kept making love to each other."

These are the gifts of loving over the course of years: a bond of devotion that lights our way, a sensuality that makes the present moment *live,* and a sexually alive lifetime of loving that leads us to the delights of being held dear for years.

One last naked thought

Being "naked" is about being transparent and honest and available to each other. It's about being willing and giving and finding ways to make our marriage more peaceful and happy. When we use the naked theme to address all of the things that promote intimacy in our marriage, what we get is ease, sweetness, and happiness.

But being naked also means being unaffected and allowing things to be simple, open, and available. For myself and my own marriage, I've found that simple is always best. Easy-to-apply shortcuts—bare and uncomplicated—work to get my husband and me into our intimacy.

We want to keep in mind that intimacy is a much broader experience than just sex. It's the ability to know each other, to discover more together as we live, to find agreement on the things that make life delightful and happy, and to build a path of strength, delight, and prowess based on those things. When we broaden our intimacy focus to include the arenas beyond sensuality, it tends to make the sex flow as well.

We want to *own* the gifts of a Naked Marriage over the course of a whole and contented life as partners. That doesn't mean we won't weather hard and even grievous things as we walk this earth. We will. But we also get to claim life's joys—the sweetness of its gifts offered up to us—and the wonder of a deepening love.

All we need to do is to step up and claim it.

A Naked Marriage is meaningful in the best sense of the word; it's good, kind, enriching, momentous, deep, and enlivening. It's real and true and wholly worth the effort. And we deserve every drop of the luscious marital elixir of love that we can muster. *Every drop.*

To take those early sparks we felt for each other—the quirky, amazing electricity of them—and build something *mature* upon them over years is our gift, and it is also our charge. We want to be willing to throw out the idea that a passionate marriage should look like our early dating life and instead get our hands and bodies into the adult stuff of *loving over time.*

The handful of strategies in this book help make intimacy work. They help us *insist* upon our loving, hold it, keep it, and build upon it.

Once we start practicing these suggestions, their gifts become so clear and so straightforward that it's nose-on-our-faces obvious: we work into our hearts and bodies a regular wakeup call that gets us skin to skin and opens us up to desire, sex, and sensuality. We build prowess with each other by having set-aside, uninterrupted time for our sex life. We learn easy affection and time-out for romance together. We create agreement and simple communication strategies, learning to listen and share with each other regularly. We get some agreement with our lifestyle and money choices so they don't block our desire. We find the place where closeness lives and dwell in it.

On our ninetieth birthdays—if we're still kicking—we will know for sure that we've had a true and world-altering love affair that has been with us through all of life's normal, crazy, and challenging stuff.

That's the power of the Naked Marriage. Closeness. Intimacy. Sensuality. Desire. Accessibility. Ease. Joy. Love. All right here for the taking.

ACKNOWLEDGMENTS

I must absolutely thank Brooke Rockwell, my superb editor (and now friend) who offered her terrific expertise with humor, grace, and delight all through this process. To the amazing team at Skyhorse—particularly to Leah Zarra—thank you, from my heart, for being on-your-game, as well as being so responsive and expert. It is truly a pleasure to work with you.

I owe a deep debt of gratitude to my agent, Joelle Delbourgo, whose vision, determination, and commitment to *Naked Marriage* made it lift off the page, and who found the best home for it. Joelle: to be believed in, guided, and honestly supported is a great gift to an author, and you have gone above and beyond the call.

My thanks also to Herb Schaffner and Laura Schenone of Big Fish Media, fine friends and wonderful writer/editors who offered early and mid-course shaping of the manuscript, and did it with enthusiasm and love for the written word.

I offer a resounding cheer of thanks to every one of the couples and individuals who offered their intimate experiences to me, so that this book might really help other couples: it was a personal and giving act, and I am grateful.

Lastly—and with all my body and soul—I thank my husband, Michael Nagler, who loves me, stands by me, champions my work, and steers me in the right direction when I am going off the track, and who I adore beyond measure. I thank you, Michael, for being brave enough to encourage me tell the truth about our own intimate experiences, so that others might find the grounded-in-joy sensuality that we've found. You're the best thing that ever happened to me, by far.